A MINUTE FOR
YOUR HEALTH!

A MINUTE FOR YOUR HEALTH!

―――――⚬∿⚬―――――

THE ABC'S FOR IMPROVED
HEALTH AND LONGEVITY

Edited for

The Association of Black Cardiologists, Inc.

by Stephanie H. Kong, M.D.

2005 Edition—Revised and Updated

HILTON PUBLISHING COMPANY • CHICAGO, ILLINOIS

Hilton Publishing Company
Chicago, IL

Direct all correspondence to:
Hilton Publishing Company
110 Ridge Road
Munster, IN 46321
815–885–1070
www.hiltonpub.com

ISBN 0-9764443-0-5

Library of Congress Cataloging-in-Publication Data

Kong, Stephanie H.
    A minute for your health! : the ABC's for improved health and longevity / edited for the Association of Black Cardiologists, Inc. by Stephanie H. Kong.—2005 ed., rev. & updated.
        p. cm.
    Includes bibliographical references and index.
    ISBN 0-9764443-0-5 (pbk. : alk. paper)
    1. Longevity. 2. Health. 3. Nutrition. 4. African American physicians. I. Association of Black Cardiologists. II. Title.
    RA776.75.K66 2005
    613.2—dc22   2005017314

Printed and bound in the United States of America.

CONTENTS

ରେ

Section I: Practical Guidance For Health, Well-Being And Longevity

ର

Section IV: Living With Heart Disease

ର

Section V: Practical Guidance For Women, Pregnant Moms And New Moms

༖

Section VI: The Role Of Mental Health On Longevity

༖

Section VII: Lifestyles That Shorten Your Life

ବ

Section VIII: Living With The Big "C"

ବ

Section IX: Take A Minute For Your Lungs

ବ

Section X: Take A Minute To Learn About Common Medical Problems

ABOUT THE EDITOR AND THE ASSOCIATION OF BLACK CARDIOLOGISTS, INC.

Stephanie H. Kong, M.D.

In addition to the clinical practice of medicine, Dr. Stephanie Kong has dedicated her career to improving the health of African Americans by developing strategies to empower adults to take control of their health and motivate others to do likewise. As a Pediatric Resident at Milwaukee Children's Hospital, she authored a practical guide for mothers, "Hey Mom, Did you Know?", which emphasized active participation of mothers in the health of their children. Dr. Kong has spent most of her professional career as a managed care executive. She has served on the clinical faculty of the Medical College of Wisconsin, Penn State- Hershey Medical Center and The Johns Hopkins University School of Medicine. She has authored several publications on managed care, quality of life, and preventive medicine. She is currently the Chair of the Cultural Competence Committee of the Association of Black Cardiologists and resides in Atlanta. She and her husband, Dr. Waine Kong, have four children (Jillian, Freddy, Melanie, and Aleron) and three grandchildren (MacKenzie, Brooks, and Audrey).

The Association of Black Cardiologists, Inc.

The ABC was founded at the first CVD disparities conference in the United States by 17 progressive cardiologists and scientists at the American Heart Association annual meeting in Dallas, Texas in 1974. They dedicated the organization to reducing the cardiovascular disease burden in the African-American community. The original intent was to partner with government, industry, foundations, churches and professional organizations as well as to make membership available to all who are concerned about the reduced life expectancy and heart health of African Americans.

The American Heart Association provided staff support (Mr. Glen Bennett), and Dr. Richard Allen Williams, our founder, served as President for the first twelve years. In 1986, the by-laws were changed, Dr. B. Waine Kong was hired as the Chief Executive Officer, and a succession of incredibly innovative presidents (Drs. Daniel Savage, Elijah Saunders, Jay Brown, Augustus Grant, Paul Douglass, Frank James, Elizabeth Ofili, Malcolm Taylor, and Paul Underwood) contributed to the success of the organization and the reduction of heart disease, diabetes, and stroke in our community.

With the recognition that by age 21, due to cardiovascular disease, African-American children are fortunate if they have one surviving grandparent, in 1997, the ABC adopted the mantra "Children Should Know Their Grandparents so they will become GREAT Grandparents Themselves." This slogan has galvanized the community and solidified our commitment to reducing our susceptibility to cardiovascular disease. If we want to meet those wonderful people in our future, we must take better care of ourselves today.

In order to improve the quality of life and longevity for African Americans, the ABC promotes:

- The development of culturally competent health care providers.
- Equal access to medical care and innovative technologies.
- Greater access to African-American physicians, specialists and other health professionals.
- Preventive, holistic health with our recommended seven steps to good health.

NOTE FROM THE EDITOR

I am so pleased to provide you with the second edition of A *Minute for Your Health*. The first edition was so widely and well received that through an additional education grant from Pfizer Medical Humanities Initiative, the Association of Black Cardiologists, Inc., was able to revise and to provide additional "minutes" that can assist you, the reader with practical ways to help you and your family maintain healthy lifestyles.

Over the past twenty years, in my role as wife, mother, grandmother, pediatrician and managed care executive, I have become convinced that we don't need to spend more dollars on health care and medicine; what we need to do is 1) think more about our bodies and our health each day, 2) adopt life styles that promote health and not disease, 3) be honest with ourselves and the physicians we are in partnership with to cure disease when it occurs and 4) be prudent shoppers when it comes to selecting a physician, a hospital or an insurance company. As quiet as it is kept, YOU, the consumer, are the most important part of the healthcare continuum. Disease and health starts with YOU—without disease there would be no need for 1) hospitals, physicians, medicines, 2) the insurance companies that pay for the hospitals, physicians and medicines from the premiums you paid or tax dollars you paid, 3) the lawyers who sue the hospitals, doctors and pharmaceuticals companies when you are dissatisfied or get worse and not better, or 4) the government officials that regulate this $1.4 trillion dollar medical-health industry. DISEASE IS BIG BUSINESS and WITHOUT YOU, DISEASE COULDN'T HAPPEN! WOW!

Now, am I saying that all diseases are completely preventable? Well, of course not. What I *am* saying, however, is that the diseases that are the most common reasons that shorten your life and decrease the quality of your life can be prevented. You don't have to have a heart attack from high blood pressure, obesity, or diabetes. You don't have to have a premature baby if you take care of yourself during pregnancy. You don't have to have a stroke if you reduce your blood pressure. You don't have to get infected with HIV or die from AIDS if you practice safe sex. Remember you are promised three score and ten years, which is 70 years of life! Many of us never reach that promise because we shave the years off by promoting a disease-prone lifestyle by not taking better care of ourselves. There is no magic pill for youth, longevity, or a disease-free life. There is a prescription, however, if followed, that can enhance the quality of your life and add years to your life. The TIPS found in this book are part of the prescription; regular church attendance along with a positive outlook on life is another portion.

Live each day to the fullest and to the best of your ability by taking a *Minute for Your Health* each and every day.

With my warmest and heart felt regards and thanks. Here's to your health!

Stephanie Hisako Kong, M.D.

FOREWORD

Dale A. Matthews, M.D., F.A.C.P.

*Associate Professor of Medicine, Georgetown University School of
Medicine, Washington, D.C.*

*Author, The Faith Factor: Proof of the Healing Power of Prayer (N.Y.,
Viking, 1998)*

*The fear of the LORD is the beginning of wisdom and knowledge of the
Holy One is understanding. For through me your days will be many and
years will be added to your life.*

            ᠗ Proverbs 9:10–11, NIV

Since the days of Solomon, the wise have recognized that religious
commitment and reverence for God helps us keep up our physical,
emotional, and spiritual health. Authentic faith, as the Bible defines
it, means, "being sure of what we hope for and certain of what we do
not see" (Hebrews 11:1, NIV). People who have that kind of faith are
less likely to develop medical and mental illnesses or to abuse drugs
and alcohol. They are more likely to recover from medical illnesses
and surgery. The faithful also tend to have a higher quality of life,
which includes strong marriage and satisfaction with one's job and
one's life in general. When our lives are grounded in such ways, we
have a better chance of staying healthy, or, if we get ill, making a
strong recovery.

Perhaps for that reason, religious people tend to live longer than
people who aren't religious. The faithful are less likely to engage in
risky behavior, and more likely to follow physicians' advice and to
engage in healthy behavior, such as exercising, eating a healthy diet,
and wearing seatbelts. This thoughtful care for themselves stems
from the high value and satisfaction they find in their lives, and their
determination to treat the body as the temple God gave them.

Why does religion strengthen our powers to heal, and even protect us from falling ill? In *The Faith Factor: Proof of the Healing Power of Prayer* (Viking, 1998), I give some answers. Religious practice:

- lessens the likelihood of depression and strengthens our ability to cope with the stresses in our lives.
- reduces drug and alcohol use, and increases our willingness to work with doctors and other health care providers.
- brings renewed spiritual energy through the beneficial role of adoration, worship, confession, repentance, and forgiveness.

Another way that religion benefits us is that it provides us with social support. Worshiping with people to whom we are bound in community, by shared beliefs, rituals, sorrows, and joys, can be a powerful source of personal support. It can help us through our own illnesses, by reminding us that our community is pulling for us, body and soul. And in times of serious illness or bereavement, our spiritual community can ease the demands and burdens on us and create an atmosphere that supports healing.

The community itself can thus become a mediator and an instrument of healing, and open the path for divine intervention. It can help us hold in mind that an infinite God desires the healing of each individual regardless of race or social situation. You will remember the desperate man, ostracized from his society because of his leprosy, who broke through an astonished crowd and fell on his knees before Jesus, beseeching him, "If you are willing, you can make me clean!" And you'll remember the outcome. Jesus said, "I am willing. Be clean!" and the leper was healed (Mark 1:40–41). That story testifies that the compassionate heart of God intends healing for all persons.

The apostle Paul writes, "your body is a temple of the Holy Spirit, who is in you. You are not your own; you were bought at a price. Therefore, honor God with your body." (1 Corinthians 6:19–20). This book will help individuals and congregations honor God not only with worship but also with greater determination to treat the body as a temple of the Holy Spirit.

The Association of Black Cardiologists has been a national leader in recognizing the important role that minority congregations can play in preserving and strengthening the individual and collective health of its members. The trust and esteem the church enjoys in the African-American community has helped promote better health for Black Americans–a project very badly needed.

A *Minute for Your Health*, intended for distribution as part of weekly programs of worship, recognizes the unique importance of the Black church in enhancing the health of African Americans. While we are among the most deeply religious groups in the United States, too many of us have poorer health and less access to care than other Americans. Each chapter addresses one important health concern that is relevant to the needs of a congregation.

These brief chapters can't cover everything, but each raises an issue that can be discussed more fully by the congregation's health professionals and clergy, either as part of weekly worship services or through fellowship or educational meetings. Health tips provided by A *Minute for Your Health* can be included in your church bulletin. Such information can help close the unfortunate and unnecessary racial gap readily obvious in health statistics today. By reading and discussing these health tips with your family and friends you can help spread the good news.

A MESSAGE FROM THE PRESIDENT OF THE ASSOCIATION OF BLACK CARDIOLOGISTS, INC.

The A *Minute for Your Health* project began in 1988 when Rev. Nathaniel Johnson of the Mount Moriah Baptist Church in York, PA asked Dr. Stephanie Kong to give brief health-related messages during Sunday morning services. In Rev. Johnson's words, "I want this congregation to be the most knowledgeable and the most healthy in Pennsylvania." In addition to these brief oral health messages, Dr. Kong wrote and published them in the church bulletin so church members could later refer to them.

The Kongs left York, Pennsylvania in 1991 and relocated in Sacramento, California where Dr. Kong continued this work; she had these messages published weekly in the *Sacramento Observer* and she encouraged churches to clip these weekly messages and reprint them in their church bulletin.

In 1995, after moving to Atlanta and realizing that these health-related sound bites were well received, Dr. Kong offered them to the ABC and A *Minute for Your Health* was published for the first time under the auspices of the Community Health Risk Reduction Program Committee of the Association of Black Cardiologists. The objective of each message was to give a minute's worth of health information that members of church congregations could readily understand, accept, and use. Ms. Jackie German, who was the Director of Community Programs, helped to prepare the first "Minute for your Health" primer, and was particularly instrumental in securing the support of Dr. Dale Mathews, who wrote the forward.

As you will soon discover, this book is not just about heart disease, diabetes, and stroke. Although these are major area of concerns for the Association of Black Cardiologists, we thought it was also important to provide guidance in other areas of health so that our patients, our congregants, and peers could begin their journey with the Seven Steps to Good Health:

- Be Spiritually Active
- Take Charge of Your Blood Pressure
- Control Your Cholesterol
- Track Your Blood Sugar
- Eat smart and Enjoy Regular Exercise
- Don't Smoke
- Access Excellent Healthcare and Take Medications as Prescribed

All of us have tasted the bitter fruit of one of our loved ones leaving us too soon due to a stroke or a heart attack. Such deaths are shocking to those left to mourn, because often we were not aware until too late that our loved one was ill. This lack of awareness of potential health problems is particularly common in the African-American community.

By consciously reading all the messages, you will be amazed how a little bit of information will impact on your overall health and well being. We tend to ignore symptoms because of denial, fear, or mistrust of the health care industry. Black patients, especially men, often come for help only when their condition is at an advanced stage and treatment is no longer likely to provide a satisfactory result.

If we are to improve the health of African Americans, and Americans in general, we must all work together. As it is, too many of the people whose strength and experience we sorely need are cut down prematurely by weakening, sickness or death. When this happens, our young people miss opportunities to share the experience of wise elders. The result is that too often the young repeat the mistakes of their parents, instead of being guided to better lives by the wisdom of their elders.

It was my pleasure to invite Dr. Kong to serve as editor for this edition, and a heart felt thanks goes to Pfizer Medical Humanities Initiative for providing the funding for this iteration of "A Minute for

Your Health." We hope you enjoy the improvements and updates of the information. Some of the material was adopted from publications from the ABC Epidemiology Center edited by Ms. Melanie Dowdell, Ms. Marcia Sutherland, Chief Financial Officer for the ABC, was an invaluable proofreader.

A *Minute for Your Health* provides a series of health tips that, through study and discussion, can break bad health habits that weaken our community. By spreading the word in your congregation and the community at large, to your family and your friends, you can make a difference that matters profoundly to us as a people.

Prevention and early diagnosis are the keys to good health. Each of us should be the bearer of that good news.

We hope you enjoy this monograph and equally hope that through the application of the health messages you will ensure that your children know their grandchildren so that they will become GREAT grandparents.

Paul Underwood, M.D., President,
Association of Black Cardiologists, Inc.

THE POWER OF ONE MINUTE

Mike Magee, M.D.

Director, Pfizer Medical Humanities Initiative
Vice President, Pfizer Science and Medical Advocacy

Can a minute make a difference?

When the Pfizer Medical Humanities Initiative partnered with the Association of Black Cardiologists (ABC) in 2003 to create the previous edition of A *Minute for Your Health*, we were betting it could just take a minute. The 75 health tips in the book might each only take about a minute for you to read, but if put into practice, they could help add years to your life.

Readers responded to this vital information in an easy-to-digest format, and demand for the book surpassed all expectations. Two years later, we are happy to help ABC bring you this new expanded edition of A *Minute for Your Health*, with 110 health tips on topics ranging from healthy diet to cardiovascular disease to health insurance.

We hope you'll share A *Minute for Your Health* with others through religious and community organizations. Use this book to inform and empower yourself, your family, your friends, and your neighbors. Some of the biggest killers—including some diseases like stroke, heart disease, diabetes, and HIV that disproportionately affect African-Americans—are highly preventable. Health awareness is a crucial part of a healthier community.

Mike Magee, MD

INTRODUCTION

Again the word of the Lord came to me, saying, "Son of man, speak to the children of your people, and say to them: 'When I bring the sword upon a land, and the people of the land take a man from their territory and make him their watchman,

 'When he sees the sword coming upon the land, if he blows the trumpet and warns the people, then whoever hears the sound of the trumpet and does not take warning, if the sword comes and takes him away, his blood shall be on his own head.

 'He heard the sound of the trumpet, but did not take warning; his blood shall be upon himself. But he who takes warning will save his life.

 'But if the watchman sees the sword coming and does not blow the trumpet, and the people are not warned, and the sword comes and takes any person from among them, he is taken away in his iniquity; but his blood I will require at the watchman's hand.'

 "So you, son of man: I have made you a watchman for the house of Israel; therefore you shall hear a word from My mouth and warn them for Me."

꙳ Ezekiel 33:1–7

Today, heart attacks, diabetes, strokes, and other cardiovascular diseases continue to lead the nation's top causes of death. In addition, diseases such as HIV/AIDS, tuberculosis, and hepatitis keep spreading, despite our best efforts to stop them. The tragic fact is that for African Americans, all these diseases take an especially high toll because these diseases are the grim reapers that steal our grandfathers and grandmothers from our communities and in doing so, destroy the storehouses of knowledge, love and understanding housed in them. When a grandparent dies, an entire library goes up in flames.

For people of faith, challenges and even tragedies are best met when we can turn our burdens over to God, and find strength in his blessings and grace. The challenge is to improve the health of our people.

Ezekiel 33:1-7 powerfully explains the role of the watchman. If as watchmen, we see each other suffering and dying from disease and poor health, it is our duty to alert and educate one another, and, in that way, help prevent the pestilence.

Each of us must first hear the watchman, and follow his warning that we improve our diets, lifestyles and behaviors. But each of us must also *become* the watchman, by sounding the trumpet to alert and ultimately help others. If our brothers and sisters succeed in finding and keeping their good health, we succeed; if they fail, we fail. The burden of ill health rests upon each of us. We *are* our brothers' keepers!

It is my hope that a physician, nurse, dentist, or other health professional will share these messages weekly with a congregation. The messages may be read aloud as part of the service, printed in the church bulletin, or both. We believe that this program is non-intrusive, and at the same time, reinforces the advice of the member's own physician. It is a simple idea that can significantly improve our collective health status.

"You don't have to be sick to get better." Most Americans today know what will keep them healthy and what's likely to make them ill. The difficult part is getting people to make this information work for them. For instance, most of us know that

- Smoking will increase our risk of heart disease, cancer and emphysema, but one out of six of us continue to smoke.
- Too much animal fat in our diets will clog our arteries, but we continue to eat hot dogs, hamburgers, bacon, and doughnuts. These doughnuts add too much sugar to our diet—and too much sugar in the blood can lead to obesity and diabetes.

- Too much alcohol will ruin our livers, our relationships, and increase our rate of accidents, but many of us continue to drink too much and at the wrong times.
- Seat belts can save our lives in an accident, if we wear them regularly.
- High blood pressure and elevated cholesterol increase our chance of stroke and heart disease, but one out of three of those affected with these health risks do not have them under medical control. Nor do people realize how one baby aspirin a day can help in this control.

I hope that these messages will help move your congregation toward greater health awareness, and help move members and their families toward changes that will make them healthier, stronger, less likely to fall ill, and more likely to recover if they *do*. The messages are offered in the spirit of health ministry, as lessons that may help our children know their great grandparents.

The message to get from "Healthy People 2010" is *Heal Thy People*.

Stephanie H. Kong, M.D.,
Editor

For more information on any of the issues highlighted in this book, please write to:

B. Waine Kong, Ph.D., J.D.,
Chief Executive Officer
Association of Black Cardiologists, Inc.
5351 Hunter Road
Atlanta, GA 30349
800–753–9222

You may also visit our website: www.abcardio.org

SECTION 1

---❧---

PRACTICAL GUIDANCE
FOR HEALTH, WELL-BEING
AND LONGEVITY

1. CHILDREN SHOULD KNOW THEIR GRANDPARENTS SO THEY WILL BECOME GREAT GRANDPARENTS

But Jesus Said, "Suffer little children, and forbid them not, to come unto me: for of such is the kingdom of heaven."

ବ୍ୟ Matthew 19:14

Grandparents are a national treasure and resource. Grandparents are libraries filled with knowledge, love, and experience. Our "libraries" are dying off too soon and with them all the wealth of information that can be passed on. If we are ever going to solve our social problems, we need grandparents to live longer, healthier lives. We need grandparents to be available to their grandchildren. Think of a community free of juvenile delinquency, adolescent and unwanted pregnancies, school dropouts and under-achievement. These communities can be realized through the influence of grandparents. A child is only a grandparent away from developing into happy, well-adjusted, contributing members of society. Children readily defy their parents, but they think twice about upsetting grandma or grandpa. There's authority that children respect.

Grandchildren are also fun. In fact, one grandmother said, if she knew that grand children were going to be so much fun, she would have had them first! Your grandchildren are your legacy and your immortality. After all is said and done, what you leave behind are your children and their children's children. So, treat them well. Tell them the stories. Teach them to pray and to be respectful. And make sure you continue to be available to them.

So why are so many of our "libraries" closing down? The problem is that due to heart disease, diabetes and stroke, too many grandparents leave us even before their grandchildren arrive. This is the thief that is robbing African-American children of their grandparents. Cardiovascular disease kills more than half of all grandparents—more than all the other causes of death combined. And the pitiful fact is that heart disease, diabetes and stroke is preventable. These medical conditions are lifestyle problems. How we live causes tremendous loss of lives in our fifth and sixth decades. It is not dramatic breakthroughs in medicine that will make a difference in our life expectancy. This change can only happen when we decide to take responsibility for our health and prevent disease before it happens.

As you read each health message, research the topic further either at your local public library, through the Internet or with your doctor. The secret to good health and long life lies in *your hands*. Every little bit you do will either help you a little or hurt you a little. When taken as prescribed, these health messages are the little steps to improved health that will assure that all of us become great grand-parents.

2. THE ROLE OF RELIGION IN HEALTH AND MEDICINE

Even so faith, if it hath no works, is dead.

– James 2:17

In some societies, the priest and physician are one and the same person, administering spiritual and physical healing with divine sanction; it wasn't until the 1800's that Americans began to separate medicine from religion and place more emphasis on scientific research to cure diseases. Patients, as well as physicians began to rely on science and not faith. At the same time, patients and their doctors began to emphasize the treatment of disease instead of the promotion of health.

Still, over the past several decades, there has been a broad revival of interest in spiritual healing and religious practice and health. We now recognize that the return to spirituality and religion assists our physical healing. This is accepted by most physicians. Good studies show, for example, that when patients in an intensive care unit who have had a heart attack are prayed for, they leave the hospital 3–4 days before those who have not been prayed for. On the strength of such studies, religion and spirituality have come to be considered a form of complementary medicine. In another important study, Dr. Robert Hummer, after analyzing the U.S. Household survey, came to the conclusion that African Americans who attend religious services regularly, lived on average fourteen years longer than African Americans who did not attend church.

Much of the research suggests that an active religious commitment is "beneficial for preventing mental and physical illness, improving recovery, and enhancing the ability to cope with illness." Ask any one of the "Mothers of the Church" and they will tell you that they don't need studies to confirm the power of prayer. In fact, most people who practice active prayer for healing swear by it!

4

Some of us aren't surprised to find these living connections between spirituality and healing. One of the original disciples, St. Luke, was a physician, and there are numerous accounts of Christ Himself healing the members of His audience, the relatives of His circle of friends and strangers that happened upon Him.

Along with an active spiritual life, let's all remember that God put physicians here to help us as well. As all good things come from God, He also would want us to have a positive relationship with our physician who can assist us in treating chronic diseases, such as hypertension, cholesterol and diabetes at the same time you are praying unceasingly that you maintain your health through the power of prayer. God also expects us to take care of His temple by living the kind of life that promotes health. Western medicine and faith can work hand in hand.

3. WHAT IS HEALTH?

. . . for the Lord seeth not as man seeth; for man looketh on the outward appearance, but the Lord looketh on the heart.

❦ 1 Samuel 16:7

The World Health Organization in 1948 defined Health as a "state of complete physical, mental and social well-being and not mere absence of disease or infirmity." More and more scientists and doctors includes a state of spiritual well-being as the fourth criteria that should be evaluated in health promotion. Taken together, health then becomes a state of complete physical, mental, social and spiritual well being. To be truly healthy, you have to pay attention to each aspect of your being on a daily basis.

Everyday, you should go through a checklist to ensure you have made positive strides toward your:

- Physical Health—What are the areas in your physical health that may need your attention—weight loss, control of high blood pressure and cholesterol, exercise, control of your diabetes?
- Mental Health—What are you going to do today to ensure you protect your emotions and mental health? Do you know how to think positive thoughts? Do you know how to channel your anger and disappointment? Did you laugh today? Did you give someone the benefit of the doubt? It takes less energy to be positive than to be negative.
- Social Health—What are you going to do today to interact with people and get positive feedback from people? Are you going to talk with friends? Are you going to join a group experience? Do you have a social group either at church, work or school? Isolation can lead to depression. A wise man once said, "If you have family and friends, you may stumble but you will never hit the ground." God did not mean for man to be alone. Find someone to interact with today.

- Spiritual Health—What are you going to do to feed your spiritual self today? Do you start your day with prayer or with the Word of God? The Bible says, "In the beginning was the Word, and the Word was with God and the Word was God." The spoken word is a powerful tool, whether uttered in prayer or meditation; these words fill our minds and souls and eventually become flesh in our lives. Regardless of your religious affiliation, spend some time each day in thought and meditation, not on your problems but how you can change your problems into opportunities. Christians refer to this as harnessing the power of prayer. You never get a busy signal when you call on God.

Give attention to each portion of your well being on a daily basis so that you become a well-rounded individual in positive balance, realizing your full potential.

4. FIRST AID

...for I am the Lord God that healeth thee.

ᐁ Exodus 15:26

If you don't already have a first aid kit in your house, you can make one very easily. Just follow these simple steps:

- Get a shoebox, old cookie tin, or cigar box, and clean it thoroughly. Label it clearly with the words "First Aid," and make sure every member of your family knows where you keep it.
- On the inside cover or lid, list the name and telephone numbers of your doctor, the local pharmacy, the poison control center, and the nearest hospital.
- A basic first aid kit should contain the following items:
  - Blunt scissors
  - Roll of gauze
  - Roll of adhesive tape
  - Soap
  - Bandages
  - Tongue depressor
  - Silvadene ointment (for burns)
  - Iodine
  - Peroxide
  - Syrup of Ipecac (to induce vomiting in cases of poisoning)
  - 4 x 4 gauze
  - Activated charcoal tablets (for food poisoning)
  - Tylenol

  Replenish an item when you see it is about to run out.
- One member of your family should take the Red Cross First Aid course and be trained in basic Cardio-Pulmonary Resuscitation (CPR).
- Here are some helpful first aid hints:
  - Direct pressure will stop bleeding in most cases. Also elevating the bleeding part above the heart will slow bleeding.

8

- Clean a cut, and then apply pressure or a moistened tea bag to stop the bleeding.
- If someone swallows poison, call the poison control center before giving Syrup of Ipecac.
- If you suspect that you or a loved one has broken an arm or leg, call the local Emergency Room for instructions on how to immobilize the limb and how to move the injured person.
- Put cold water or ice on a burn, and call your doctor.

No one plans to have an accident. But you *can* plan how to respond to one.

5. HOW LONG SHOULD A PERSON LIVE?

The days of our years are threescore and ten.

ஒ Psalm 90:10

The Bible suggests in Psalms 90 verse 10, that "The days of our years are threescore and ten." This adds up to 70 years. Although there has been a dramatic increase in how long the average person lives, many Americans don't live to see their 70th birthday.

Too many African Americans, especially African-American men, don't live to that biblical age. Life expectancy in the United States for White men is 74, but for African-American men it is 66. White women, on average, live to be 80, African-American women, 74. Ninety-nine percent of us still die before age 85.

In Japan, where people have the longest life expectancy, the average person lives to be 80 years old. The United States ranks seventeenth in the world in longevity even though we rank number one in terms of how much we spend for medical care. What is even more alarming is the fact that African-American men have the shortest life expectancy in the United States. In fact, men in third world countries like Jamaica and Bangladesh live longer than African-American men in the United States.

There are people who live in isolated parts of the world who have no physicians, hospitals, or synthetic drugs, and yet live longer than we do in the United States. But when they adopt Western lifestyles, they become vulnerable to diseases—the same lifestyle diseases that shorten the life of Americans.

Regardless of where and how people live, some can drink, smoke, and live dangerously, yet still live into old age. Others come into the world so weak or handicapped that they last only a few days. Most of us fall within three score and ten years. But we can live longer if we keep our weight down, exercise, eat wisely, and otherwise live prudent lives. We can guarantee that our lives will be shorter if we smoke, drink too much alcohol, and fail to control our blood pressure, cholesterol and blood sugar. If you prevent disease you are likely to reach the average life expectancy. If you promote health you are likely to exceed the average.

It's your choice. Choose not to get old and die before your time.

6. DIE YOUNG AS LATE AS POSSIBLE

Say to him: 'Long life to you! Good health to you and your h household!
And good health to all that is yours!

ॐ 1 Samuel 25:5–7

Have you ever wondered why someone you know has a car that looks and acts brand new even though the car is ten years old? Or why someone else has a car less than three years old that looks and performs like a heap of junk? Could it be that the first person just took better care of this expensive property–respected it, was not reckless with it, did not drive it too fast, checked the oil, had it serviced regularly, parked it in a garage, washed it regularly, used only the right fuel, and kept the wheels from banging curbs?

The second person drove the car into the ground (six feet under). He or she did this by never taking it in to be serviced and repaired by the car doctor except when it stopped or made funny noises.

Which one of these pictures fits you?

Not only do many of us treat our cars carelessly, but we also treat our bodies the same way. We don't take our cars in for routine maintenance and don't take the time to do the same thing for ourselves. You've probably heard a friend say, "I can't live without my car." The question your friend needs to ask is: "How well would I live without my body?"

Far too many of us become disabled, get old, or die before our time. We carelessly eat, drink, and smoke, do not exercise, do not see a doctor when we should, and do not follow the doctor's recommendations when we do see one. In the end, we rob God, ourselves, our families, our church, and our communities of an invaluable asset that can't be replaced–ourselves.

It's true that with the human body, as with a car, the product you start with can make a big difference. In most cases, a BMW will last longer than a Chevy, given equal treatment. Similarly, people who are born with good genes are likely to last and stay strong longer than people with bad ones. But most of us come into the world some- where in between—not with genes that will keep us going no mat- ter how badly we take care of our bodies, and not with genes that will destroy us even if we take the best of care. That's why prevention–taking good care of yourself and seeing a doctor regu- larly–is so crucial to your health and longevity.

At his 90th birthday party, Eubie Blake once said, "If I had known I was going to live this long, I would have taken better care of myself."

7. MORE PREVENTION—LESS TREATMENT

. . . for a man's life consisteth not in the abundance of the things which he possesseth.

ᕋ Luke 12:15

Imagine that life is a mountain road that all of us must travel. Because many of us like to live on the edge, from time to time, some of us will fall off the precipice and hurt ourselves. The response in Western society is to develop a very sophisticated system to respond to our pain and suffering. In the US, we have a wonderful ambulance system, trained emergency personnel, great hospitals, physicians and surgeons who will pick you up and try to put you back together again. Wouldn't it make sense to try to prevent the fall in the first place? What if we just put up some barriers along the way?

There are models in Western medicine that relied more on prevention than cure to tackle a widespread problem. The problem was tooth decay. Not long ago, everyone expected to gradually replace his or her natural teeth with false teeth. Many of us even remember toothaches. Dentists mostly pulled teeth and dental labs were busy making false teeth. Clinicians and scientists provided the answer. They made three recommendations:

- Fluoridate our drinking water
- Brush and floss our teeth twice a day
- See the dentist twice a year for check-ups, not just when you have a toothache

It worked! Ninety percent of Americans born in the last forty years will now die with our natural teeth, the denture labs are mostly gone and most dentists now do other procedures than pulling teeth. Our children have never had a toothache. Most of the diseases that plague us are preventable and under our control, we just need to adopt a preventive orientation to life. We can and should prevent bad decisions, debts, unhealthy relationships and disease. We should control the amount of stress in our lives.

If we get used to the idea that it is a good idea to prevent the problem or illness rather than to try to treat it after falling off the "disease cliff." We will live a long time and enjoy a great quality of life. It is very difficult to put Humpty Dumpty together again after a great fall.

As your first step toward prevention as a lifestyle, embrace these "Seven Steps to Good Health" promoted by the Association of Black Cardiologists:

- Be Spiritually Active
- Take Charge Of Your Blood Pressure
- Control Your Cholesterol
- Track Your Blood Glucose
- Eat Smart and Enjoy Regular Exercise
- Don't Smoke
- Access Excellent Healthcare and take Medications as Prescribed.

8. PREVENTION IS CHEAPER THAN CURE

If thou wilt diligently hearken to the voice of the Lord thy God, and wilt do that which is right in his sight, and wilt give ear to his commandments, and keep all his statutes, I will put none of these diseases upon thee.

ᘒ Exodus 15:26

If you were living one hundred or more years ago, you would be concerned about dying from such diseases as cholera, typhoid, small pox, tuberculosis, scurvy, beriberi and rickets. Today, because of improved nutrition and sanitation, we no longer have to worry about those diseases. Instead, we die of diseases that are a direct result of our "improved" standard of living, such diseases as:

- Heart attacks
- Strokes
- Cancer
- Accidents
- AIDS
- Cirrhosis of the liver
- Diabetes.

Many of these are preventable. Today, we're likely to live twice as long as we would if we had been born a hundred years ago. We owe this longer life span to several breakthroughs in knowledge and understanding:

- Our political leaders helped by cleaning up our sewage systems, purifying our water, and disposing of our garbage.
- Nutritionists taught us more about healthy diets
- Modern medicine taught us about contagious diseases and how to prevent them from spreading
- The church taught us "Cleanliness is next to Godliness"

Modern medicine has probably taken us as far as it can. We enter a new century where good health depends more and more on the choices we make. If we want to live longer and to improve the quality of our lives, we must learn to prevent diseases rather than seek cures after we get sick.

Changing the way we live is the best way to prevent disease. The first step is to identify the risk factors in our own lives and take steps to correct them. So here are a few questions you need to ask yourself:

- Are you overweight?
- Do you smoke?
- Do you exercise?
- Do you drink alcohol excessively?
- Do you use illegal street drugs?
- Do you eat too much salt and animal fat?
- Do you eat a lot of sugar?
- Do you drink too much coffee?
- Do you drive recklessly?
- Do you have unsafe sex?

If the answer to any of the above is yes, take stock of yourself and make a change. You are shortening your life and may not experience the full richness of life that is available to you.

Accept the facts: you *are* the master of your body and tomorrow *is* the first day of the rest of your life. When it comes to maintaining your health, you have to be responsible for yourself. You must recognize that there is a cause and effect relationship between what you do and how long you live. Once you have learned to act on this, you can begin to teach it to others.

Let us approach tomorrow not in quiet desperation, but with gusto, each of us fully responsible for our fellow man and for ourselves.

9. RECIPE FOR HEALTHY LIVING

For we walk by faith, not by sight.

ଡ଼ 2 Corinthians 5:7

Here's a simple recipe to promote a healthy lifestyle. If you practice these steps you will experience the fullness and richness in life we all seek:

- 1 ounce of prevention (much better than a pound of cure)
- 5 servings of fruits and vegetables per day
- 8 glasses of water
- ¹/₂ dozen good friends (relatives are OK as well)
- 30 minutes of exercise per day
- 4 cups of laughter (no substitutions)
- 1 mustard seed of faith
- 2 tablespoons of patience (add more if you have children)

Add a dash of adventure (fun can be substituted, but increase the amount). Also add a bunch of love (enough to share). Mix well and live long.

The following ingredients are known to ruin the recipe:

- Couch potatoes
- Excessive alcohol
- Smoking
- Stress
- Negative thinking
- Negative attitudes
- Excessive fats and sugars in your diet
- A complaining attitude or spirit
- An unforgiving spirit
- No social interaction

A wise man once said, " as a man thinks, so is he!" Truer words were never spoken. What you put into your vessel will bear fruit so make sure that our vessel is getting health ingredients daily.

10. THE TIES THAT BIND—THE FAMILY AND ITS IMPORTANCE

And walk in love, as Christ also hath loved us, and hath given Himself as an offering.

                                        ⓢ Ephesians 5:2

For a while, when it seemed that America was moving too fast, people stopped talking about the fundamental importance of family values. Today, many of us view the family unit as the best way to promote the mental and physical health of each family member, and to promote stable and well-adjusted children. That consensus has become a movement. If you wish to be part of this movement, here are some steps you can take to strengthen your family.

Step 1: *Make sure everyone in your family knows that your family comes first.* Mr. Spock of *Star Trek* once said, "The needs of the many outweigh the needs of the one." Everyone in your family unit should know that parents will promote the interests of the family as well as the interest of each family member. As children grow up, they need the assurance that their projects and interests are as important as work responsibilities. Promoting everyone's importance will ensure that each member of the family will promote the "Family First" idea. A wise man once said, "If you have family, friends, and God, you may get tripped up or stumble, but you will never hit the ground."

Step 2: *Promote each other's individuality.* In promoting the family unit, it's also okay to want to become an individual with interests outside of the family unit. The family becomes the "safe haven" that everyone can retreat to, while learning to be individuals with their own particular strengths and weaknesses.

Step 3: *Promote joint decision-making.* When conflicts arise, it's important that the family get together to discuss the problems and solutions. An ideal family get-together is one where people can say what they really feel, without fear of reprisal. Some families set aside Thursdays as the day the family gets together to discuss individual and collective challenges. During these weekly meetings, the children and parents could discuss tough issues—with the ground rules being 1) no criticism and 2) everyone promoting problem solving and not laying blame. Whatever method is used, families should set aside specific times to discuss important decisions and problems, with everyone's understanding that although a democratic process is being promoted, the final decisions will rest with parents.

Step 4: *Never give families members the broken cookies.* A lot of families put aside the "good" stuff, like the best cuts of meats or unbroken cookies, for company and not family. When company came over to your house when you were a kid, maybe your mother would break out the fine china. Maybe you even wondered why you weren't able to eat off of the fine china. Such behavior is usually justified along the lines that it is always good to put your best foot forward for company. Well, perhaps we need to put our best foot forward for our families first.

Step 5: *Teach adaptability and an ability to roll with the punches.* There are no set rules that can govern what families will experience in our uncertain times. Financial and occupational successes and failures can occur overnight. Children often can sense that something is not right and perhaps you as the parent are under stress. Not sharing the problem with the child doesn't prevent the child from sensing that something is wrong and sometimes the lack of knowing is more damaging than the crisis itself. Children have imaginations and can imagine the worst. Clue your children in on your problem solving skills so that they can see success in real time as you begin to unravel your challenge through solid and calculated decision making. If the family has to make certain sacrifices, share the reasons with your children so that they truly are a part of the solution and not the problem.

Step 6: *Have a Thirsty Ear*: When family members are experiencing difficulties or significant events in their lives, all family members can participate by listening. That's a way of assuring the person who needs your support that you care and that their issue is important to you and worth listening to. When you are acknowledged and listened to by the people you consider special in your life, you can't help but feel special and draw strength from their love and support.

Step 7: *Teach social responsibility.* A wise prophet once said, "To whom much is given, much is expected." Every family should encourage its participants to give to each other and to give back to society in a meaningful way. The world could benefit from more of us sharing our talents and skills. Teach your children to be volunteers. Every person in America, regardless of economic circumstance, should know the value of volunteerism. Martin Luther King once said, "We can all be great, because we can all serve."

Step 8: *Promote a spiritual life for the family and individual members of the family.* A family that prays together, stays together. God created the family unit as a reflection of His love, nurturing, and expansion of humankind. Promote family prayer and church-going even during those tough years when you have teenagers who believe they have all the answers. One day they will wake up and realize how smart you were as parents. The scripture says, "Train up a child in the way he should go; and when he is old, he will not depart from it."

Step 9: *Make family time sacred.* Whatever time is set aside daily or weekly for family interactions or gatherings, that time should be protected and kept sacred. Turn off the phones, television and anything else that will detract from the quality of interactions during your family time. Members of families should not miss graduations, birthday parties, family reunions, weddings, births and deaths. Just think, your family is the only evidence that you walked this earth. Your family is your legacy.

Step 10: *Make grandparents part of the nuclear family.* Strong families value the participation of grandparents and other extended family members. Grandparents have the time to be good listeners and advisors. In a forest, only those trees with deep roots ever grow tall enough to reach the sun!

11. DO YOU HAVE A LIVING WILL AND AN ADVANCE DIRECTIVE?

A good man leaves an inheritance for his children's children

෴ Proverbs 13:22

A Health Care Advance Directive or Living Will is a document in which you can give instructions about your health care if, in the future, you cannot speak for yourself. You can give a family member or friend the power to make health care decisions for you if you cannot make them for yourself. You can also give instructions about the kind of medical care you want or don't want in the event you are incapacitated.

There is a difference between a Living Will and a Health Care Advance Directive. In a traditional Living Will, you state your wishes about whether you want life-sustaining medical treatments if you are terminally ill. In an Advance Directive you direct your own care through instructions you leave, and appoint someone else to make medical treatment decisions for you if you cannot make them for yourself.

If you cannot make or communicate decisions because of a temporary or permanent illness or injury, a Health Care Advance Directive helps you keep control over health care decisions that are important to you. In your Health Care Advance Directive, you state your wishes about any aspect of your health care—including decisions about life-sustaining treatment—and choose a person to make and communicate these decisions for you.

It's important to have an Advance Directive before you need it because, unless you formally write out your instructions and appoint someone to decide for you, many health care providers and institutions will make critical decisions for you that might not be based on your wishes. In some situations, a court may have to appoint a guardian.

An Advance Directive also can relieve family stress. By expressing your wishes in advance, you help family or friends who might otherwise struggle to decide on their own what you would want done. Be assured that a Health care Advance Directive only kicks in if you are unable to make your own decisions.

Every state has laws that permit individuals to sign documents stating their wishes about health care decisions when they cannot speak for themselves. The specifics of these laws vary, but the basic principle of listening to the patient's wishes is the same everywhere. The law gives great weight to any form of written directive. If the courts become involved, they usually try to follow the patient's stated values and preferences. A Health Care Advance Directive is the most convincing evidence of your wishes.

You should immediately do two things:

- Appoint someone as your Agent.
- Write out instructions for your care.

Stay in control of your own health care! Make your wishes known while you are able.

12. WHAT IS A RISK FACTOR?

For if ye forgive men their trespasses, your heavenly Father will also for-
give you. But if ye forgive not men their trespasses, neither will your
Father forgive your trespasses.

လ Matthew 6: 14–15

A risk factor is like running a red light: sometimes you can get away
with it, but eventually you are either going to get hit or at least get a
ticket.

There are specific risk factors for each disease that afflicts
humans. A risk factor is a condition that makes it more likely you
will come down with a particular disease. Here are some examples:

- Participating in un-safe sexual practices can lead to sexually
  transmitted diseases such as syphilis, gonorrhea, HIV-AIDS,
  and unwanted pregnancy.
- If you don't brush your teeth, or you allow babies to sleep with
  bottles in their mouths, you have increased the risk of developing tooth decay.
- Not washing your hands after you sneeze or use the bathroom
  is a risk factor in spreading diseases.
- Smoking is a risk factor in causing lung cancer and heart disease.
- Not getting your baby shots increases the risk of developing
  childhood diseases like whooping cough, measles and mumps.

Whatever the disease, there are known risk factors that, if avoided,
can lead to a healthier, longer life.

Cardiovascular risk factors are those factors that increase the
likelihood of your dying at a young age from a heart attack, congestive heart failure or stroke. The heart and vascular system are
affected by risk factors such as being overweight, having diabetes, not
exercising or having hypertension. These risk factors are completely
controllable by you without you having to go to expensive gyms, having expensive operations or being on constant diets.

Obesity and diabetes are the greatest risks of ensuring that you will not live long enough to enjoy your grandchildren. Sixty percent of Americans are overweight and another twenty-seven percent are morbidly obese, meaning they are over a hundred pounds over-weight. When you pack on that kind of weight, the fat is stored not only under your skin, but also in your muscles—including your heart muscle and in your blood vessels. Your heart and blood vessels can't function the way they were intended to under this increased strain, therefore they suffer damage (heart attacks, brain attacks, and strokes).

Obesity is also a risk factor for the development of diabetes. More and more of our teenagers are obese and therefore develop cardiovascular diseases in their fourth and fifth decades of life. Diabetes can cause your kidneys to fail, your heart to fail and even-tually you to fail.

Both obesity and diabetes are preventable so why are Americans continuing their cycle of destruction by eating themselves to death? Americans spend $100 million dollars per year eating at fast food restaurants and then spend another $30 million dollars trying to lose weight.

The secret to weight loss is simple. You have to burn more calo-ries than you consume. If you want to consume 3,000 calories a day (double the recommended daily caloric intake) you have to make sure you are going to burn 3,000 calories a day. If you don't then you have gained weight that day. Every three cans of soda, 3 bags of potato chips or a single slice of pizza will add a pound of fat to your body. See how simple it is to take control of your life!

Diets do not work. Follow three simple rules:

- Reduce portion size . . . no seconds.
- Reduce sugars. In other words, avoid sodas, cookies, dough-nuts, and cakes; do not have sugar in your home . . . get rid of the sugar bowl.
- Reduce animal fat.

If you eat a lot, exercise a lot. But remember, you must run one mile to burn off the calories of one hot dog.

Take a minute to write down the health conditions you have and then write down the risk factors next to each condition. If you don't know the risk factors for a particular condition can call your local health department, your doctor or surf the Internet. When you have listed the risk factors, implement a daily routine of attacking each risk factor. If you do that everyday, you will begin to see results. Train yourself to eat smaller portions and don't run red lights or stop signs. Just try it and see!

13. ARE YOU TAKING YOUR MEDICINE AS PRESCRIBED?

For whosoever shall keep the whole law, and yet offend in one point, he is guilty of all.

ಶ James 2:10

When your doctor prescribes medication for you, it is important that you take the dosage the doctor orders on the schedule given. Most medications have limited potency, that is, they only work for a certain amount of time. If your doctor prescribes a medication to be taken two times a day, that usually means the effect of the medication will probably only last for eight hours, so to get the full benefit, it's important that you take the medication every six hours while you are awake. You would not usually be expected to get an alarm and wake up to take your pills.

If you have a chronic disease like high cholesterol or high blood pressure, you may have to take medicines for the rest of your life. Most doctors start you with one medicine and only add more when your condition doesn't respond to just one pill. If you haven't taken the medication and your doctor doesn't know this, your doctor may be ready to add more medication, thinking the first one didn't work.

If you haven't taken your medicine, let your doctor know why; it may be that you can't afford the medicine, or the medicine makes you feel funny, weak or not yourself or it could just be that you forgot to take it. Whatever the reason, share the information with your doctor. If you can't afford your medicine, tell your doctor before you leave the office. There are programs that will allow you to purchase your medication at a very reduced rate, like the Together Rx Access card. Ask your doctor about these programs and also ask your doctor whether there are sample medications you can have.

It's also important to take antibiotics until they are all gone. If your doctor prescribed ten (10) days of a medicine and you only take it until you feel better, all you have done is killed the weak bacteria.

The stronger bacteria need the full ten days to be killed. Sometimes, when you don't kill all of the bacteria, the bacteria can attack vital organs like your heart or kidneys. So it's important that you take all the antibiotic medication as prescribed for you.

If you have a question about the medication prescribed for you, get an answer from your doctor or the nurse. Once you have the information you need, you are more likely to be comfortable with the medication. Invest in your health and take the medication prescribed for you.

SECTION II

———— ⚬⚬ ————

THE BUSINESS OF
MEDICINE AND HEALTH

14. HAVING A MEDICAL HOME

*And thou shalt teach them diligently unto thy children, and shalt talk of
them when thou sittest in thine house, and when thou walkest by the
way, and when thou liest down, and when thou risest up."*

ꙮ Deuteronomy 6:7

None of us wants to be homeless. We need a place that gives us
refuge and love, among loved ones with whom we can share the love
that gets us through our days. But people often forget that they also
need a medical home—that is, a place where they:

- regularly receive the health care they need
- from the same caregiver or physician;
- have their medical information stored;
- trust the information being provided to them; and
- learn to do what they need to do in order to stay healthy.

Your doctor manages your medical care. Your doctor knows your
medical history, keeps records, and will alert you to any changes in
your health. But you, too, are an active partner. It is you who must
make and keep medical appointments, tell your doctor the whole
story about each illness, take your medication, and do what you
need to do to stay healthy. It is you who must know what to do in the
case of medical emergencies, or if you have an accident or fall ill. If
you have a medical home, none of this will be a mystery to you.

Another benefit offered by a medical home is that there is where
you will be given tests you need to take regularly to make sure that
your body is working as it should—tests like Pap smears, colon tests,
mammograms, cholesterol, and blood pressure checks.

Your doctor knows your medical condition and what medications you are using. Your doctor will also catch any sign of an illness
at its early stages, when it is most treatable.

Your doctor, who is your primary care provider, needs to know
all your medical history. So, if you are obliged to go to a specialist,

always request that the specialist sends a copy of the results to your primary medical home. It can be dangerous for you if one doctor is prescribing medicine without knowing what another doctor has prescribed. Sometimes you can even fail to get needed treatment because one doctor thinks the other doctor has provided it.

Remember, *"Home is where the Heart is!"* And your medical home is where your health is!

15. YOU AND YOUR DOCTOR

As every man hath received the gift, even so minister the same to another, as good stewards of the manifold grace of God.

           ဿ 1 Peter 4:10

It is up to you to have a personal physician to assist you in maintaining your health or improving your health. You and your personal physician are in a partnership that requires trust on both sides! Usually, if you take active interest in understanding your condition and treatment, that trust comes easily, out of your good questions and the conversation with your doctor that follows. If you feel that your doctor does not care about you personally, talk this over with him or her, and if that doesn't work, find another doctor.

You are entitled to know everything the doctor knows about you from your physical examination, or any tests that have been performed on you.

Doctors are more than willing to explain everything to you, if you ask.

Your trust in your doctor can also rest in the assurance that your doctor is bound by law to keep information you share with him or her confidential.

If you have to take a new medication or to be hospitalized, your doctor will probably give you the information you need to understand the treatment. If not, be sure to ask these questions:

- Why am I feeling the way I do? What do you think is wrong with me?
- What will the tests show you and what will you and I do with the results of the tests?
- Do I really need these tests? (You have a right to refuse all tests you deem unnecessary.)

- What side effects will I have with the medication that you prescribed and want me to take? (All medications have potential side effects. You may not have *any* problems with the medications your doctor wants you to take, but your doctor can predict the side effects you *might* have.)
- What risks are involved with the treatment being recommended for you?
- Do I have any options other than the treatment being recommended? (You have a right to know all your options and to choose the option that you believe is best for you.)
- How do the benefits of my treatment compare with the risks?
- How is this treatment likely to affect the quality of my life? (Beyond side effects, you should know whether your treatment affects how you feel, your memory, your sleeping patterns, as well as how well you get along with others.)
- Do I really need to be in a hospital or can I have the therapy at home? If I need to be in a hospital, how long must I stay there?
- Will I have any limitations on my activity at home? Are there things that I should or should not do, such as exercise?
- What are the signs and symptoms that I should tell the doctor immediately if they appear?
- What signs and symptoms can wait until the next office visit?

By the way, most doctors will come to your church, club, or organization to explain medical issues. You just have to ask.

The answers to these questions will put you on the road to becoming a much healthier patient. Your doctor will be happy to cooperate. This is why it's so important that you ensure that you have one medical home and that all your medical information gets there.

16. ARE POOR PEOPLE SICKER THAN RICH PEOPLE?

And Jesus answered him, the first of all the commandments [is], Hear, O Israel; The Lord our God is one Lord: And thou shalt love the Lord thy God with all thy heart, and with all thy soul, and with all thy mind, and with all thy strength: this [is] the first commandment. And the second [is] like, [namely] this, Thou shalt love thy neighbour as thyself. There is none other commandment greater than these.

ᏮᎧ Mark 12: 29–31

The simple answer to this question is YES! There is a definite relationship between your socio-economic status and your health. Poor people tend to have poorer health and tend to have illnesses that are chronic in nature. Chronic diseases such as diabetes, cholesterol, hypertension, asthma and other respiratory diseases are more common in people at or below the poverty level. The exact reason for this is unclear. However, the scientists and policy makers think it has something to do with the fact that if you are poor you may not be able to:

- Have regular doctor visits.
- Purchase all the medications you need.
- Eat a balanced diet.
- Reduce the stress in your life.

People who live in poverty are also affected at a higher rate by lifestyles practices such as unsafe sex which can lead to HIV infection and AIDS, smoking which can lead to cancer, drug use which leads to a generalized poor health status, low exercise rate which will lead to joint disease and obesity and eating a lot of sugars and fats which will lead to diabetes and hypertension.

Also, if you are poor and African American, your health is the WORST of the WORST! A big reason why African Americans, especially those living in the South, are the sicker portion of the U.S.

population is due to the fact that some physicians do not care for African Americans aggressively and appropriately. If you are an African American with heart disease, you may not be referred by your doctor to have a cardiac evaluation by a specialist. If you are an African American with hypertension, your doctor may not prescribe the right drugs for you. If you are African American, your doctor may not evaluate if you have kidney damage from your hypertension. These are facts and you have to be part of the solution.

Here are some simple steps you can take to ensure that you are receiving the best care:

- If you are over 40 and have had hypertension for more than five years, ask your doctor when he or she will be sending you to a specialist to make sure that your heart and kidneys are okay.
- If you have hypertension, and see a cardiologist, ask the cardiologist when he or she will test how well your heart is working.
- If you have diabetes, ask you doctor when he or she will be testing your hemoglobin A1–C and when your kidneys and your eyesight will be tested.
- Make sure you get Pap smears at least on a yearly basis.
- Make sure you are taught to do breast self-examinations and if you are over 40, start having mammograms.
- Make sure you are on the right medications. Some medicines for hypertension and heart disease work better than others in African Americans.
- Ask your doctor about the best diet and exercise plan for you.
- Take the time to know your doctor and make sure your doctor knows you.
- When you change doctors, make sure your new doctor knows about all your chronic illnesses and the surgeries you have had.
- If you don't have health insurance, ask your State Medicaid Department for the locations of Federally Qualified Health Centers in your area. If there are none, then your County Hospital will be able to provide care for you and let you pay what you can afford.

- Avoid using emergency rooms unless you have a true emergency. It is better to have your health care delivered by a clinic or a physician who knows you.

The relationship you have with your doctor should be open and honest and could save your life.

17. MANAGED CARE AND YOU

He that is void of wisdom despiseth his neighbor: but a man of understanding holdeth his peace.

᠖ Proverbs, 11: 12

You owe it to yourself to understand managed care so that you can maximize your benefits. First, what managed care is not. Managed care is not an attempt to ration care or withhold care from consumers. Managed care companies are required by law to approve and pay for all medically necessary services that are listed as benefits in your contract with them.

In order for managed care to work for you, you as the consumer must be aware that:

- Your employer, Medicaid, or Medicare, has made a decision concerning benefits to which you are entitled. It is your responsibility to know what coverage has been purchased on your behalf. You must also understand that the managed care company will pay only for those benefits that have been purchased for you by your employer, Medicaid, or Medicare. For example, you and your doctor may feel that you need cosmetic surgery. Cosmetic surgery is usually not a covered benefit that your employer, Medicaid, or Medicare pays for. Therefore, the managed care company will not authorize you to receive cosmetic surgery. On the other hand, if the benefit you seek *has* been provided as a covered benefit, then the managed care company must authorize you to have that benefit if the services you seek are medically necessary.

It is your responsibility to know what coverage has been purchased on your behalf.

- It is the responsibility of you and your physician to determine with the managed care company whether the services you seek

37

are medically necessary. Often, the outcome will hinge on whether, in your doctor's view, you require a special test or medical procedure to help diagnose or treat your medical problem. Sometimes simpler tests or further observation of your condition is what is needed, rather than an expensive test or surgical procedure. On the other hand, such tests may prove to the managed care company that the more expensive test or procedure *is* needed.

- When you receive services from a physician other than your personal physician, be sure that this physician has a contract with your Health Maintenance Organization. When a physician is contracted, you can be sure that his or her credentials are good and that you will not receive a bill for the services performed. When you receive care from non-contracted physicians (outside the network), you will usually be responsible for payment of the service even when you are a member of the HMO.

Although managed care organizations have many rules and can be a hassle, the benefit to you is to limit what you have to spend from your pocket for health care. This is especially true if you need ongoing medication or medical care. Used properly, with a right understanding on your part of the rules of the game, managed care can work for you.

18. HOW AND WHEN TO GET A SECOND OPINION

And Pharaoh said unto Joseph, I have dreamed a dream, and [there is] none that can interpret it: and I have heard say of thee, [that] thou canst understand a dream to interpret it. And Joseph answered Pharaoh, saying, [It is] not in me: God shall give Pharaoh an answer of peace.

ဤ Genesis 41: 15–16

There are always two people interacting in your health care. YOU and your health care provider or physician. Physicians are human beings just like you and they come in all different sizes, shades, and shapes. Even though they, for the most part, all wear white coats, physicians and other health care providers are just as much a product of their upbringing and environment as you are. Also, even though their training can be similar, health care providers have their own opinions and experiences. Some health care providers take a more conservative, or traditional, approach, while other health care providers are more aggressive and tend to use the newest tests therapies even in corporate alternative medicines. Since health care (including mental health) is highly specialized and constantly changing, it can be difficult for every health care provider to be skilled in the latest technology.

Most physicians don't mind if you ask for a second opinion because this also helps the physician to get more information. Sometimes getting a second opinion from a different health care provider might give you a fresh perspective and more information on how to treat your condition. You can then weigh your options and make a more informed choice about what to do. If you are given similar opinions from two health care providers, you also can talk with a third heath care provider. The main point is that you have to be in charge of your health and medical care. Just like Joseph in the passage above, the physician is there to provide guidance and suggestions, but it takes you to execute the plan of action.

Here are some tips for how to get a second opinion:

- **Remember that a competent physician or health care provider never gets upset when you ask for a second opinion.** If your physician or health care provider gets upset when you ask for a second opinion, perhaps you should change providers. When it comes to your health, the last thing on your mind should be whether or not you are hurting your physician's feelings.
- **Ask your physician or health care provider to recommend a specialist for another opinion.** Don't worry about hurting your physician's or healthcare provider's feelings. Most physicians or health care providers welcome a second opinion, especially when surgery or long-term treatment is involved.
- **If you don't feel comfortable asking your physician or health care providers about whom to go to for a second opinion, contact another healthcare provider or physician you trust.** You can also call medical societies like the Association of Black Cardiologists, university teaching hospitals, and medical societies in your area for names of physicians or health care providers who deal with your particular medical problem. Some of this information is available on the Internet.
- **Always check with your health insurance provider first to make sure they will cover the cost of a second opinion.** Many health insurance providers do. Ask if there are any special procedures you or your primary care doctor need to follow.
- **Arrange to have your medical records sent to the second opinion physician or health care provider before your visit.** This gives the new physician or health care provider time to look at your records and can help you to avoid repeating medical tests. You need to give written permission to your current physician or health care provider to forward any records or test results. You can also request a copy of your medical record for your own files. The medical records belong to you!
- **Learn as much as you can about your condition.** Ask your physician or health care provider for information you can read,

go to a local library, or do a search on the Internet. Some teaching hospitals and universities have medical libraries that are open to the public. But, be aware that sorting through information that is complicated and sometimes contradictory can be a daunting task. List your questions and concerns and bring the list to discuss with the physician or health care provider you are seeing for a second opinion.

- **Never rely solely on the telephone or Internet for a second opinion.** When you get a second opinion, you need to be seen by a physician or health care provider. A sound second opinion includes a physical examination and a thorough review of your medical records. Don't forget to ask the physician or health care provider to send a written report to your primary physician and get a copy for your records.

19. THE MEDICARE PRESCRIPTION PROGRAM

But strong meat belongeth to them that are of full age, [even] those who by reason of use have their senses exercised to discern both good and evil.

ᐁ Hebrews 5:14

This new coverage is known as Medicare Part D. It is also called Medicare prescription drug coverage. It is open to all people with Medicare, regardless of income. People with Medicare will soon have to make decisions about this coverage. So if you have Medicare, it is important to know what it means for you. Even if you have a prescription drug plan now, this program may help you more.

Medicare prescription drug coverage starts January 1, 2006. It can help you. It's coverage you can depend on.

- It's open to everyone on Medicare. If you qualify for Medicare, you can join. Your income or the condition of your health will not matter.
- It helps protect you from high drug costs. You will have peace of mind knowing that you will be covered even if you have high drug costs.
- It's easy to get the facts. Call 1-800-MEDICARE (1-800-633-4227). TTY users should call 1-877-486-2048. Or you can visit www.medicare.gov.

Here's How Medicare Prescription Drug Coverage Works
- You can choose from at least 2 Medicare prescription drug plans in your area.
- If your income is limited and you have few assets, you may be able to get extra help from Medicare. Then you won't have premiums or deductibles to pay. You will have lower co-pays as well.
  - Extra help is available if your annual income is below $14,355 for a single person or $19,245 for a couple *and* if

your assets are under $11,500 for a single person or under $23,000 for a couple. People who qualify or may qualify for this help should get a letter from the government. Read this letter closely. Learn about your choices.

- Most people will pay around $37 per month. You will also pay for the first $250 of your drug costs per year.
- After that, Medicare will pay for 75% of your drug costs up to $2,250 per year.
- You will pay for all drug costs between $2,250 and $5,100 per year.
- Over $5,100, Medicare will pick up 95% of all your yearly drug costs.
- The amounts used above represent standard coverage. Actual plans may not look exactly the same.
- Enrollment starts November 15, 2005, and ends May 15, 2006. Sign up at this time to pay a premium of around $37per month. If you are on Medicare you should sign up by May 15, 2006 or your premium may go up for every month you do not join.

This fall, look for more details in the mail from Medicare about this new program! Don't be left in the dark. Know what your options are-especially if you need to fill prescriptions regularly.

20. THE ROLE OF YOUR PHYSICIAN IN PROMOTING YOUR HEALTH

Is there no balm in Gilead; is there no physician there? Why then is not the health of the daughter of my people recovered?

ᐤ Jeremiah 8:22

Physicians undergo many years of education and training to learn about the human body and the response of the body to diseases. Physicians also spend a good deal of time and training learning about lifestyle behaviors that promote health and those that promote disease. Physicians also learn to prescribe medicines to treat disease and learn what tests to confirm a disease diagnosis.

Physicians trained in the U.S. do not, however, spend a lot of time learning about nutrition or the discipline called "preventive medicine". Physicians get even less training in learning how to persuade adults to stop risky behaviors and start those behaviors that promote health and well-being. That job is YOURS! Your physician cannot heal you or make you better. You are in charge of your health! Here are some examples:

- Your physician may correctly diagnose your high blood pressure and prescribe the correct medication. You have to get your prescription filled and then take the medicine as directed. Often medications don't work because you have not taken them appropriately.
- If you have diabetes, lipid (cholesterol) disorders, or hypertension, your physician may prescribe a new eating plan for you where you eat smaller portions, eat less saturated fat, and reduce your carbohydrates and sugars, but YOU have to follow the plan.
- Your physician may tell you to increase your exercise but YOU must exercise more.
- Your physician may ask you to return to the office in two weeks for a follow-up visit, but YOU must return.

Your physician is your guide to better health and your partner for the treatment of disease, but your health and well-being is in your hands, ultimately! Your physician is your guide to:

- A correct diagnosis.
- A comprehensive treatment plan for disease.
- Providing alternative ways in which your disease can be treated.
- Understanding the side effects of your medication.
- A schedule of preventive health visits designed just for you.
- A healthy lifestyle of eating and exercise.
- Development of a Living Will and an Advanced Medical Directive.

Your physician is your partner for better health and sound medical advice. However, the cure and prevention of disease rests squarely on your shoulders.

21. WHAT IS HEALTH INSURANCE?

And Jesus said unto him, Foxes have holes, and birds of the air [have]
nests; but the Son of man hath not where to lay [his] head.
🙖 Luke 9:58

Most Americans pay for their medical and health care bills with
health insurance. Put another way, 244 million Americans are able
to go to see a doctor, get a laboratory test or go to the hospital and
have minimal-to-no out-of-pocket costs at the time of the visit
because they have insurance. Health insurance is typically provided
through your employer or through the government. Health insurance companies are responsible for contracting with physicians and
hospitals, paying those physicians and hospitals for the care ren-
dered to you, and helping you get the care you need. On a sadder
note, 44 million Americans have no insurance, the majority of these
Americans being women and their children.

When your insurance is provided through your employer, your
employer will typically work with a "broker" to get the best coverage
for you and your family. The broker goes to many insurance companies to get the most insurance coverage for the best price.
Employers then offer this coverage to their employees and the
employee's family. The coverage costs a certain amount to be paid
from your paycheck. Sometimes, your employer will pay a portion
or all of your coverage, but if you want family coverage you have to
pay the difference. You can decide to just have yourself covered or
your whole family if you can afford it. You do not have the choice to
decide which insurance company your employer will pick unless
you have a very active union who then negotiates with the employer
to select the insurance coverage.

Sometimes employers will choose an insurance plan that costs
very little on a monthly basis; these policies usually then make you
pay more at the time of the visit, that's called the patient co-pay. That
is your financial responsibility and must be paid when you receive a
service. Some policies only begin to pay for your medical and health

care when you have spent a certain amount of money first. This is called the deductible. Again this is your financial responsibility and the insurance company will not pay any of your health care of medical service bills until the deductible is paid. Some health care policies will exclude certain conditions from coverage, such as pregnancy—if you were pregnant before you received your coverage. Check your policy for exclusions, co-payment requirements and deductibles because you are financially responsible and will get a bill from the provider even though you have coverage. Most employer-based insurance programs cover prescription medication, but you may have a high co-pay. When you have employer-based insurance, most of the time you are provided a Health Maintenance Organization option, a Preferred Provider Organization option and a Point Of Service option. Your premiums, co-payments and deductibles will vary depending on which type of coverage you chose. In any case, you are paying the premiums and therefore you're paying for a portion of the care.

Here's a tip—if you are a single Mom and you work for minimum wage, chances are, even if your employer provides you with health insurance coverage, your dependents may be eligible for Medicaid. Check with your state Medicaid office and find out if you qualify.

Medicaid and Medicare are insurance plans sponsored by the Federal Government. Medicaid is insurance for: 1) women who are pregnant and their children—if the woman meets the poverty guidelines, 2) disabled citizens who are over the age of 18, 3) nursing home coverage if you qualify by income, 4) prescription of indigents. Most states offer an HMO option for their Medicaid recipients. Most of the time if you pick the HMO option, you will get better benefits.

Medicare is the Federal insurance for the elderly. You typically have to be over 65 years of age and have paid into the Social Security system to qualify for this insurance. Medicare has three parts to it:

- Part A covers your hospital bills.
- Part B coverage pays for your doctor visits, lab tests, physical therapy and other outpatient tests. There are co-payments and

deductible requirements with Part B of Medicare. You have to pay a monthly insurance premium to Medicare to get Part B coverage.

- Starting in January 2006, those Medicare recipients with Part B coverage will be able to purchase **Part D** of Medicare and get limited pharmacy benefits. (See Chapter 19 on the New Medicare Prescription Program).

- Medicare recipients can also enroll in an HMO if they have both Part A and Part B coverage. Typically, those Medicare enrollees who chose an HMO get more benefits; some HMOs offer prescription coverage now. If you are a Medicare recipient, you may want to consider an HMO.

Just remember that "insurance" does not mean "free." You are paying for the health insurance either through your employee contribution, your taxes or through social security. Also remember that in addition to what you pay as premium, taxes or Social Security, you are also financially responsible for the co-payments and deductibles.

22. SHOULD YOUR DOCTOR LOOK LIKE YOU?

And he said unto them, Ye will surely say unto me this proverb,
Physician, heal thyself: whatsoever we have heard done in Capernaum,
do also here in thy country.

ॐ Luke 4:23

In 2001, the Institute of Medicine (IOM) published a report that stated that if you are a minority in America, especially if you are an African American, you are less likely than a White person to get needed or quality care.

The IOM's report indicated that when minorities—especially African Americans—were seen by White primary care physicians, African Americans were not as likely to be referred to heart specialists, or kidney specialists than their White patients. Nor were they referred to get the procedures to correct their coronary artery disease. African Americans were also not prescribed the correct medicines for their heart disease or kidney disease.

Now what does all this mean? Well, the answer is complex because so much of what happens between the doctor and the patient is the responsibility of *both* the patient and the physician. African-American patients are less likely to confide in White doctors. Both Black and White physicians also believe that White doctors are as likely to spend as much time with their Black patients as their white patients. The bottom line is that so much of medicine is dependent on effective communication—being able to tell the doctor what is wrong with you and the doctor being able to understand you and then helping you to get better—that the first question that each of you should ask in choosing a doctor is "Who am I more likely to communicate honestly with?"

Just as you can't be friends with everyone, not every physician you see will be the best fit for you. Just because a physician puts on a white coat, doesn't stop that physician from being human and having the same human tendencies in the exam room with you that he or she might have in a restaurant or out in the mall or in church. Remember that Martin Luther King said, "The 11 o'clock hour on Sundays remains the most segregated hour in America."

Regardless of color or ethnicity, patients who ask questions and build a relationship with their physician will get good care regardless of the color of their skin or the color of the physician's skin. As a female, I am most comfortable with African-American, female physicians. I have had very good care from male physicians and from White physicians. However, I am most comfortable with African-American female physicians because when I am communicating with my physician, she is able to relate to all of the other non-medical issues in my life that might prevent me from being as healthy as I can be.

Be a smart shopper—this is your life we are talking about. Find a physician you are comfortable with; someone you can talk to honestly and openly and then work with him or her to address those health issues and lifestyle issues that will subtract from both the quantity and quality of your life. Always remember that physicians are human and may, from time to time, have to be reminded to care for you as a total person and not just a series of diseases. If you are worried that your physician has not addressed all your concerns, then it is up to you to speak up and ask him or her to address your concerns. Jesus Christ was the only healer in written history that could tell a patient to arise and take up his bed and walk. All other mortal healers have to work with you to make your own bed and make up your mind to change those things that are preventing you from getting out of your bed and walking!

23. SHOULD YOU PARTICIPATE IN A CLINICAL TRIAL?

*And Daniel beseeched Ashpenaz to feed the others meat and wine from
the King's table but allow Shadrach, Meshach, Abednego and himself to
drink only water and eat only fruits and vegetables. At the end of ten
days, their countenance appeared fairer and fatter in flesh than all those
who ate the King's meat.*

ҩ Daniel 1: 11–15

If you have ever made up a new recipe and asked someone to try it,
you conducted an experimental trial of your recipe. When pharma-
ceutical companies think they have come up with a new treatment
or a new use for an old compound, they invite a few people to try it
before they market it to the general public. In fact, any new soap,
deodorant, eye drop, hair treatment, mouth wash or anything that
touches or enters the body must be tried on a few people before it is
permitted to be sold as safe and effective.

If you have ever been given a prescription for the treatment of
pain, blood pressure, cholesterol, arthritis, or even the common
cold, thank some volunteers who were courageous enough to first try
it before any other human being in a clinical trial. The goal of clinical trials is to find better ways to treat and help people.

Historically, mostly White men volunteer for clinical trials.
African Americans have been reluctant. Some of the reasons African
Americans are reluctant to participate may have to do with the dis-
trust of the system and the doctors conducting the clinical trial not
wanting to be treated like a "guinea pig," or just being afraid.

The Food and Drug Administration (FDA) sets very high stan-
dards of conduct for investigators and the safety of patients who volunteer. Before a drug can be "tried" in a human being, the study
must be approved by a group of community representatives and doctors who monitor the activities of the investigators and assures that
each patient is being treated as safely as possible, with dignity and

respect. You will not undergo any unnecessary or harmful tests and procedures. Most importantly, you will have every phase of the study explained to you, and an informed consent obtained before you can enroll as a volunteer.

While there can be no guarantees that participating in a clinical trial will help you, there is always a chance that you may receive the most modern and up-to-date treatment for your condition. Just like your recipe, it may be better or worse than the old dish you cooked up a long time ago. That's part of the risk of doing a clinical trial. Only you can decide if the benefits to your health are greater than the risks. So, if you are ever invited to participate in a clinical trial, at least talk to the doctor, get the facts and make an informed decision. Just remember that many other people took a chance when they participated in the clinical trials that now benefit you and your loved ones.

SECTION III

THE ROLE OF FOOD
AND YOUR HEALTH

24. WHAT YOU EAT TODAY WILL WALK AND TALK TOMORROW— AMERICANS ARE MALNOURISHED

Do not destroy the work of God for the sake of food. All things indeed are pure, but it is evil for the man who eats with offense.

                  ᘒ Romans 14: 20

How can the richest nation in the world have malnourished citizens? In some parts of the world the most visible sign of malnutrition is that people are thin and emaciated. But people who are overweight are also malnourished. *Malnourishment, simply put, is a condition in which a person is not in a good nutritional state;* more is not necessarily better!

For those of us who are overweight, the obvious solution to malnourishment is to lose weight and get to your ideal size and shape. The secret to weight loss is not dieting—it is portion size. Portion sizes are more important than what you eat! Remember, elephants and hippopotami are vegetarians—they just eat acres of vegetables a day. Pay attention to your portion size!

The human body must be in a balanced state, and this depends on how much you eat and how much physical activity you engage in. In other words, if you are overweight you must limit what you eat NO MATTER WHAT ANYONE TELLS YOU, (small portion sizes), but you must also increase the number of calories you burn through exercise. You have to be honest with yourself; if you are a PLUS SIZE person you are NOT in a positive nutritional state and you are putting yourself at risk for a life-limiting event, such as cancer, stroke, or heart disease.

Here are some helpful hints for losing weight:

- Analyze why you want to lose weight. Is it because it will help you live longer? To lower your risk of heart disease, stroke, and cancer? Or is it because you want to have more energy and feel better? Maybe your motivation is to look more attractive. In any case, you should lose weight because it makes sense to you. You'll only succeed if you're doing this because *you choose to*.

- Discuss with your doctor whether you need to lose weight and how best to do it.
- If you are overweight, you are also probably out of shape. You need to exercise. Moderate exercise is helpful **if** you do it. Don't make the excuse not to exercise because you can't jog or can't afford a gym. You can exercise at home for free and just about everyone can walk around the block.
- If you are deciding to lose weight, select a balanced diet that you can maintain.
- Examine your eating habits. Are you eating when you are not hungry because of social pressure? Or just because you see or smell food? You should eat only when you are hungry and stop eating when you are full. Limit your portion size.
- Watch less television! People who watch lots of television are tempted by the abundance of food advertisements that tempt them to nibble.
- Don't allow any food outside the kitchen and dining room. Don't eat in the bedroom, bathroom, or living room or while watching TV.
- Decide what you are going to eat before you go the grocery store, not after you buy it. If you buy it, you will eventually eat it.
- Shop for food after you have eaten, not when you are hungry.
- Drink a glass of water or eat a piece of fruit before meals. Eat slowly and eat smaller portions. Eating slowly is important because it takes 20 minutes before you *feel* full. It takes your mind that time to catch up with your body. Eat slowly and give your mind a chance to tell you that you are full.

Don't give in to the food pushers in your family. Don't let your mother tempt you with "One little piece of cake isn't going to hurt you" or "I spent the entire day preparing this for you and that's all you're going to eat?"

Remember: "What you eat today, will walk and talk tomorrow."

25. DIABETES: WHAT IS IT AND WHAT CAN I DO IF I HAVE IT?

. . . honor shall uphold the humble in spirit

ॐ *Proverbs 29:23*

Americans are overweight! Being overweight can and does cause diabetes or what the old people call "sugar". Do you remember Big Mama in the movie, *Soul Food*? Do you remember her burning her arm when she was cooking that good old' soul food, swimming in butter, grease and sugar? Do you also remember that she didn't know her arm was burning? It's because she had diabetes and one of the symptoms of having advanced diabetes is that you lose the feeling in your arms, hand, legs and feet because of poor circulation. Mama eventually died in the movie because of uncontrolled diabetes.

Diabetes happens when the sugar you eat stays in your blood stream and is not carried into the cells of your organs. Your organs-your brain, your heart, your kidneys, your blood vessels-require sugar to do their work. If the sugar stays in the blood, the blood gets too thick and your brain tells you to drink water to dilute your blood. That's why people with diabetes are usually thirsty and have to urinate a lot. You have to move sugar from the blood to the cells, which is the role of insulin. Your body only makes a certain quantity of insulin. When we eat too much sugar there isn't enough insulin to move the sugar from the blood to the cells, which is why if you are diabetic, your doctor will put you on insulin. However, the insulin you take as a shot is not as good as the insulin your body makes, and unless you cut down on the sugar you eat, taking insulin will not help you to protect your organs. It is much better to control your dietary intake of sugar whether you have diabetes or not.

In fact, 30 million Americans are either being diagnosed with, or on the verge of being diagnosed with, type 2 diabetes as a direct result of overeating. So many Americans are developing diabetes that this disease was declared by the Centers for Disease Control as the "epidemic of our time." If this trend continues, the rate of diabetes will increase by 165 percent by 2050. There is hope, however, because even modest lifestyle changes can prevent the onset of the disease or help to control its progression to kidney failure, amputations, blindness, impotence, heart disease, stroke, and death. Diabetes is the seventh leading cause of death and 80 percent of patients with diabetes die from heart disease or stroke.

You don't have to run five miles per day or starve yourself to prevent diabetes. The common sense way is just to reduce your portion sizes and the number of calories you take in. Put another way, you can get into better shape by reducing your diet by one can of soda or a bag of French fries or potato chips - or by walking a mile per day. This will translate into a better quality of life and a longer life.

It turns out that the difference between a normal person who is not prone to diabetes and an overweight person who predictably develops diabetes is 150 calories per day—the same calories in a can of soda (sugar water)! Just eating a little less or being a little more active will reduce your risk of type 2 diabetes if it is done consistently.

If you develop diabetes, it can be controlled. Consider Halle Berry. She has diabetes but is also in great shape. However, more diabetics end up as Mama did in *Soul Food*. Let's work together to control the growth of diabetes in our lifetime.

26. WHAT IS THE HEMOGLOBIN A1C TEST?

. . . for I have learned, in whatsoever state I am, therewith to be content.
                            ℘ Philippians 4:11

If you have diabetes, you need to make sure your doctor is ordering the Hemoglobin A1C test for you at least four times a year. People with diabetes check their blood several times a day by pricking their fingers, drawing a drop of blood, and using a small glucose meter to measure the sugar level in the drop of blood. This sugar level tells you what is happening with your blood glucose or blood sugar at the time you are measuring it, but it doesn't tell you what your average blood sugar was for the past three months. The Hemoglobin A1C test, by establishing the average over a 90–day cycle, lets your doctor see how well you have been managing your blood sugar. In other words, your glucose test is a pop quiz and the Hemoglobin A1C is a semester exam!

Here's a chart that you can keep with you to tell you how well you are doing with your Hemoglobin A1C.

Hemoglobin A1c	Levels	Blood Sugar Level
14	Seriously elevated levels	360
13		330
12	————————	300
11		270
10	Elevated Levels	240
9	————————	210
8	Slightly elevated	180
7		150
6	————————	120
5	Non diabetic levels	90
4		60

Remember, when you expose your blood vessels and organs to high levels of sugar for long periods of time, you damage the wall lining to the blood vessels. Damaged blood vessels can leak, causing a hemorrhage or can be the site for plaque formation, which may close the vessel. This can lead to strokes, blindness, amputations or heart attack. Having a high Hemoglobin A1C means you have had high levels of sugar floating around for a while.

The Hemoglobin A1C test is the best way to tell how well you are doing at controlling your glucose and insulin levels. If you get a result of seven or less, you are probably doing well.

27. YOU ARE WHAT YOU EAT

Whether therefore you eat or drink or whatever you do, do all to the glory of God.

> ❧ 1 Corinthians 10:31

People who live off their own land and most people in underdeveloped countries have to do a lot of physical labor to get enough to eat. For them, it's no problem burning off everything they eat.

For some of us, however, going to the supermarket is as much physical work as we do. To make matters worse, many Americans also overeat and do not live in a way that burns off calories.

It doesn't matter what the latest diet fad says; the basic indisputable rule of obesity is, if we eat more calories than we burn up, the extra calories will turn into fat.

If you like to eat, exercise more, burn up the calories. If you do not like to exercise, eat less.

Most of us eat too much, and the more we eat, the more we seem to need and want. Few of us work hard enough to burn up what we consume. If you insist on eating too much fat, sugar, salt, and calories, you will pay a price. Some foods, like fats, have more calories than other foods. For example, a cup of fat or sugar has twice as many calories as a cup of fruit or vegetables. People sometimes believe that they can't get fat because they are vegetarians. But remember, elephants and hippos are vegetarians.

A calorie is a calorie and it does not matter where it comes from. Most overweight women can lose a pound per week by limiting their calories to 1500 calories a day. Most overweight men can do the same on 1800 calories per day. Just imagine yourself with fifty pounds less weight in just one year. Of course, this also works the other way. If you only gain two pounds per year for twenty years, you will be forty pounds heavier.

To get all the nutrients your body needs, carefully follow a food plan that your doctor or dietician recommends.

The hardest part of any weight loss plan is to admit that your eating habits must change if you want to lose weight. If you can't accept that fact, get comfortable with the likelihood that you will live a shorter, less healthy, and, perhaps, less fulfilling life.

28. HEALTHY EATING LEADS TO A HEALTHY LIFE

And whatsoever ye do in word or deed, do all in the name of the Lord Jesus . . ."

                     ᎧᏅ Colossians 3:17

Two out of three people will die from heart disease or cancer. Eating too much fat contributes to both. Most Americans, even slim ones, eat too much fat. Why take the risk? It is time you discovered how delicious low-fat, low-sugar eating can be.

Here are some guidelines for reducing the fat in your diet:

- Listen to your body and eat only when you are hungry and stop when you are full—no matter how good the food is. It is better to dump excess food that to overstuff your body.
- Learn to say "No" to your mother and all the other fat-chefs and food pushers in your life. They will find other ways to show their affection for you than feeding you to death. Maybe the time will come when you can show *your* affection by leading them toward a healthier diet.
- Find better ways to handle stress than overeating. Take a brisk walk when you feel a binge coming on. You'll find it refreshing, and you'll lose weight.
- Avoid red meats and eat more fish, fresh turkey and chicken-without the skin and visible fat. But because extra fat and salt are usually added to processed turkey and chicken, a vegetarian diet is even healthier.
- Use olive, canola, or safflower oils for your gravies when you fry or sauté. Avoid lard, butter, coconut and palm oils.
- A serving of fruit or raw vegetables before meals will help to fill you up with good stuff and leave less room for the bad stuff. When you feel that you absolutely have to eat something sweet, try low-fat yogurt, sherbet, sorbet, Jell-O, Italian ice, or pudding made with skim milk.

- Avoid eggnog, mayonnaise, salad dressing, whole milk and cream. Save your two eggs per week for Saturday morning. When you drink milk, make it skim milk, and when you eat cheese, make it low-fat, such as cottage cheese, mozzarella, or ricotta.
- Avoid pastries, doughnuts, and croissants. Eat whole grain bread, English muffins, bagels, pretzels and breadsticks. Beans (legumes) and cereals are good substitutes for nuts and processed flour.
- Avoid sausages, scrapple, bacon, hot dogs, hamburgers, and lunchmeats such as corned beef and pastrami.
- Boil, broil, steam, bake and roast, instead of frying.

If you follow these ten commandments, you will look better, feel better and live longer.

29. READ THE LABEL

As for these four children, God gave them knowledge and skill in all learning and wisdom: and Daniel had understanding in all visions and dreams.

                                      ᐁ Daniel 1:17

If you buy it, somebody is going to eat it. So you need to know exactly what you're putting into your own or your family's shopping cart. Knowing the nutritional value of a particular food, along with ingredients that could be harmful, is quite easy. Thanks to the Food and Drug Administration, the label on the container of every packaged food you buy lists all the ingredients in order. By reading the label, you can avoid foods that are bad for you and enjoy delicious *and* nutritious foods that do you good.

The label lists the ingredients in their order by weight. If water is listed first, as in juices and soft drinks, that means there is more water in it than anything else. If sugar or fat is listed first, there are more of these than anything else.

For practice, compare the nutritional content of whole milk to that of skim milk or low-fat milk. A serving of whole milk has 150 calories while a serving of low fat milk has only 89 calories but 30 percent of those calories will be from fat. Both types of milk have the same nutrients except for the fat. (Incidentally, in spite of its name, buttermilk is low in fat and calories because it gets its thickness from acidification, not from butter.)

Besides telling you all the ingredients, the label lists the percent of the recommended dietary allowance contained in each ingredient, and the types and amounts of fat contained. Finally, the label gives the serving size, serving per container, as well as the number of calories per serving.

When the label says, "May contain one or more of the following ingredients" and then lists several oils, it means that the manufacturer had the option of using any of those oils in the product–including coconut and palm oil, which are especially high in fat.

Compare similar products and buy those with the lowest fats and sugars.

The FDA has no official definition of "natural," "low cholesterol," "light," "lean," or "low-fat," but food manufacturers like to use them, often in a confusing way. "Natural" does not mean that the ingredients are healthful or that dietary experts approve of them. "All-natural ice cream" may contain coconut oil that can raise your cholesterol. Foods low in cholesterol may be high in calories. "Lean" may mean fewer calories but more fats.

Sugars and sweeteners are the most common food additives in American foods and come in many forms–such as dextrose, corn syrup, maltose, and even molasses. Salt is easier to detect because it always has "sodium" in the name–such as sodium bicarbonate or mono-sodium glutamate (MSG).

You may not be able to control what goes into your mind but you can be careful about what you eat.

30. THE FACTS ABOUT FATS

Study to show thyself approved unto God, a workman that needeth not to be ashamed, rightly dividing the word of truth.

∾ 2 Timothy 2:15

All fats are divided into saturated, polyunsaturated and monounsaturated fats, in different proportions. Saturated fats, or "bad fats," come mostly from meat and dairy products. Coconut and palm kernel oils are also saturated. These fats raise your cholesterol and clog your arteries. You can recognize them easily because they harden at room temperature.

Less than ten percent of what you eat should come from saturated fats. Saturated fats are commonly found in whole milk, cheese, butter, cream, beef, pork, lamb, and poultry skin.

Marketers of prepared foods high in saturated fats can advertise that they are cholesterol free even if they use coconut and palm oils. But these saturated fats are converted to cholesterol by your body. The truth about coconut and palm oils is that they are naturally high in saturated fat and you should avoid them.

Once you have reduced the total intake of fats and cholesterol, fine-tune your diet by replacing saturated fats with monounsaturated fats such as olive, canola and peanut oils.

We all have trouble remembering which fats are which, and which are the good, which the bad. So think of "Poly" and "Mono," the good sisters, and "Sat," the bad sister. Polyunsaturated fats are the good fats, which do not harden at room temperature. These include safflower, sunflower, corn, soybean, and cottonseed oils. Also included in this group are fish oils like cod liver oil. Polyunsaturated fats are better for cooking than saturated fats that come from animal fats and tropical oils. There is even better cooking fat called olive oil, a monounsaturated fat.

There are two types of polyunsaturated fats. Omega-6 fats are the vegetable oils and Omega-3 fats are the fish oils. Whether fat or lean, fish is among the healthiest of meats you can choose. Lean fish comes from either fresh or salt water like catfish, trout, perch, and bass and have little or no Omega-3 fatty acids. But while they don't give you the good fats, they don't give you the bad ones either. Fatty fish usually comes from the deep sea and contains high amounts of Omega-3 fatty acids, which are good for you. The fish highest in Omega-3 fatty acids are sardines, salmon, mackerel and herring.

One warning: Shrimp and lobster, actually contain more cholesterol than most meats.

Except for that, next time you go grocery shopping, "go fish."

31. "YE ARE THE SALT OF THE EARTH"

If your brother is grieved because of your food, you are no longer walking in love. Do not destroy with your food the one for whom Christ died.

&ª Romans 14:15

Salt. This four-letter word packs a punch. It has been used as currency. Man has fought wars over it. Gandhi's resistance to British Rule over India began in resistance to Britain's control of salt.

Why is this substance, so vital to our health, suddenly controversial in our own time? The controversy began when nutritionists learned that by eating less salt we can reduce the risks of water retention and high blood pressure.

The fact is, we now put salt into just about everything we eat and drink. This means, you are often getting heavy doses of salt without even knowing it. That's how this simple mineral that started out as a preservative of food and therefore life, has become a potential danger for millions of Americans.

Salt contains sodium, one of the "essential elements" that we must eat to survive. Like most other things, if we eat too much of it, it becomes a problem. Too much salt in your body may cause your body to hold on to some of the water it should get rid of. If you have too much water in your system, your blood pressure may go up.

One out of ten of us is said to be "salt sensitive," which means we are more likely to have problems with water retention. Be mindful of the many ways we get excess sodium added to our diet—for example, from:

- Baking soda in baked and canned goods
- Flavor enhancers in canned vegetables
- Meat tenderizers

Learn to cut down the amount of salt in your own kitchen and on your table. Try substituting garlic, lemon juice, pepper, vinegar and other spices on your shelf. Experiment and try some of those strange-sounding and mysterious spices like paprika, ginger and sweet basil. You may just like it. In fact, salt substitutes are also high in potassium, an element of which we need more. Since most of us do not eat enough potassium, this is another good reason to try salt substitutes.

32. INCREASING POTASSIUM IN YOUR DIET

My son, attend to my words; incline thine ear unto my sayings. Let them not depart from thine eyes; keep them in the midst of thine heart. For they are life unto those that find them, and health to all their flesh.

～ Proverbs 4:20–22

Americans eat too much salt and not enough potassium. For good health, we need to keep these two minerals in balance. Potassium helps the muscles maintain their strength. It is also needed by each cell so the body can do its job efficiently.

Vomiting, diarrhea and certain medications for hypertension, especially water pills (diuretics), will lower the blood potassium. Low potassium may cause general weakness, (especially in the leg muscles), cramps, and irregular or abnormal heartbeats. A study done at Cambridge University in England found that eating more potassium could reduce the risk of stroke-related deaths by up to 40 percent.

Foods rich in potassium include fish, chicken, beef, beans, green vegetables, and all fruits. Bananas, prunes, cantaloupe, grapefruit, oranges, melons, molasses, potato skins, and berries are particularly good sources. Sun-dried fruits such as raisins, dates, figs, apricots, and prunes are low in sodium and high in potassium—good stuff!

If you overcook these foods or even just let them sit in water for a long time, the potassium will leach out into the water. If you overcook your vegetables, you will have to drink the "pot liquor" to recover the potassium!

33. UNDERSTANDING CHOLESTEROL

We are to be "living sacrifices," holy and pleasing to God–this is our spiritual act of worship. We should also be transformed by the renewing of the mind.

ᴓ Romans 12:1–2

We all have cholesterol in our blood. Cholesterol is produced by the liver, and it is necessary to the body because it is part of the outer lining of the cells. But if your cholesterol level gets too high, cholesterol can interfere with the circulation of your blood and cause heart problems. If your total cholesterol level does get high, your LDL is too high (greater than 80) and your HDL is too low (lower than 960), then you need treatment, which is simple and effective and has very few side effects.

Unlike some other dangerous conditions, high cholesterol in itself doesn't cause pain or make you feel tired, weak, or sick. But if you don't do something about it, it can lead to a heart attack or stroke.

If everyone in the United States reduced their total cholesterol by 20 percent, the number of heart attacks would decrease by 40 percent per year.

You can easily find out if you have high blood cholesterol by having a blood test. If your level is high, you can lower it by exercising and changing the kind of food you eat. The most concentrated sources of cholesterol are egg yolks, donuts, and organ meats. A diet high in fatty meats and whole milk products stimulates cholesterol production by the liver.

Some people have to take medicine to reduce the amount of cholesterol in their blood. But most people can lower it to safe levels by just lowering the saturated fat in their diet. Remember, the knife most likely to kill you is a butter knife!

71

34. LDL-CHOLESTEROL:
THE BAD GUYS

And thou shalt bind them for a sign upon thine hand, and they shall be as frontlets between thine eyes. And thou shalt write them upon the posts of thy house, and on thy gates.

ᐸᴗ Deuteronomy 6:8–9

The bad guy of the cholesterol world is LDL-cholesterol. Cholesterol is transported in the blood in little packages called *lipoproteins*. Cholesterol transported by low-density lipoproteins (LDL) is bad for you. Cholesterol transported by high-density proteins (HDL) is good for you. When you have too much LDL cholesterol moving around in the blood, it spreads like poured concrete, making a layer of gooey stuff inside the walls of the blood vessels. This gooey stuff mixes with other substances to form plaque–a thick, hard, coating that can clog the arteries, especially the small vessels that deliver blood to the heart. The process is called *atherosclerosis*.

The more plaque in the arteries, the greater your risk of having a heart attack, because this garbage may eventually completely clog up the arteries. Elevated LDL cholesterol is considered a reliable predictor of a heart attack. If your LDL number is more than 100 mg/dl, it is too high. It is best to maintain it below 80 mg/dl. The lower the number, the lower your risk of heart attacks.

In order to reduce your LDL-cholesterol, eat more fruits and vegetables and reduce egg yolks, red meat, donuts, and dairy products. And be sure to have your doctor check your LDL levels once a year.

35. HDL-CHOLESTEROL:
THE GOOD GUYS

We are vessels of His mercy which He has prepared beforehand for glory.
 Romans 9:23

If you've ever played Pac-Man, you've enjoyed watching the little head eat up the little dots. HDL-cholesterol gobbles up cholesterol from blood vessel walls just like Pac-Man, and delivers it to the liver where it is discarded. It picks up the garbage like a good sanitation worker. A high level of HDL-cholesterol protects against a heart attack. The opposite is also true—a low level of HDL increases your risk of a heart attack. Levels less than 35mg/dl contribute to the highest risk and levels above 60mg/dl are associated with the lowest risk. The higher the better.

Smoking, being overweight, and not getting enough exercise all contribute to lower levels of HDL-cholesterol. Smokers can increase their HDL by just stopping their habit. Other ways of increasing the HDL include eating a healthier diet, losing weight, and exercising regularly.

Women have protection from heart attack until menopause because they usually have high HDL-cholesterol.

36. THE DIFFERENCE BETWEEN CHOLESTEROL AND FATS

Death and life are in the power of the tongue: and they that love it shall eat the fruit thereof.

☙ Proverbs 18:21

A food that contains no cholesterol may contain lots of fat. Cholesterol comes only from animal products. But although vegetable shortening, avocado, peanut butter, nuts and coconut oil have no cholesterol, they contain a lot of fat. When you eat too much saturated fat, wherever it comes from, the body converts some of it into cholesterol.

You can help keep your HDL levels high and the LDL levels low by paying attention to the fats you take in. There are three types of fats:

- Saturated fats, or bad fats, come from animals, coconut and palm oils. They harden at room temperature and stimulate the liver to make more LDL-cholesterol.
- Polyunsaturated fats, or good fats, do not harden at room temperature, and include safflower, sunflower, corn, soybean, and cottonseed oils. When we substitute these good fats for saturated fat in the diet, the liver makes less LDL-cholesterol.
- Monounsaturated fats, the best fats, include olive oil, peanut and canola oil. Oils in this group are good for us because when we substitute these for saturated fat they will increase HDL, the good cholesterol.

For good health and long life, keep your LDL low and your HDL high!

---

37. OVEREATING IN CHILDREN

Wherefore be ye not unwise, but understanding what the will of the Lord is. And be not drunk with wine, wherein is excess; but be filled with the spirit.

☙ Ephesians 5:17–18

There is a silent predator—call it the obesity demon—that is making our children fat and unhealthy. Nearly 25 percent of our children ages 6 to 19 years are overweight. Thirty years ago only 4 percent of our children were overweight. Being overweight puts our kids at increased risk of heart disease from high cholesterol and high blood pressure. It puts them at risk for type 2 diabetes, which was previously considered an adult disease, kidney disease, and some forms of cancer. Just as important, the most immediate consequence of being overweight is that our children develop poor self-esteem and depression.

Obesity in children and adolescents is generally caused by lack of physical activity, unhealthy eating patterns, or a combination of the two. Genetics can also play a role in determining a child's weight. But let's concentrate on the lifestyle issues, since they are the ones we can change and remedy.

Our society has become very sedentary. Television, computer and video games contribute to our childrens' inactive lifestyles. Forty-three percent of adolescents watch more than two hours of television each day. Children, especially girls, become less active as they move through adolescence. Schools have cut out physical education, and only a few children participate in organized sports. Schools have chosen to put soda and candy machines and fast food restaurants on their premises to pay for needed equipment and books, which further compounds the vicious obesity cycle. Also, more and more families are turning to fasts foods for breakfast, lunch and dinner to meet the demands of women working outside of the home and having the responsibilities of family life. African-American children often eat high sugar foods (donuts and sodas) for breakfast instead of balanced meals from the five food groups. Lack of a balanced meal can make children hyper-active and malnourished.

If your child is overweight, here are some helpful hints:

- Take your child to the doctor to be examined and to define the amount of weight that is desirable to lose.
- Let your child know he or she is loved and appreciated whatever their weight.
- Increase the amount of physical exercise your child gets. Make sure your child is physically active. It is recommended that children get 30 minutes of physical activity per day.
- Plan family activities that provide everyone with exercise that is fun. Children love games and dancing, but resist "exercise."
- Make sure your child starts out with a balanced breakfast. Breakfast is the most important meal of the day and, when balanced, will have protein, carbohydrates, dairy products and grain. The reason for this is simple—breakfast literally means BREAK-THE FAST from the night before. Your brain needs fuel 24 hours a day and when you are sleeping you are obviously not eating, so your brain and other vital organs have to turn other fuels into sugars. The stored sugars get burned first, then fats and then proteins. A child who eats these three food groups in the morning will have the sugars when the proteins kick in at about 10 or 11 o'clock in the morning when he or she needs to think in school. Kids who only eat sugars for breakfast will not have that boost from their morning meal and will experience "the sugar lows" right around the time the proteins should be kicking in. Arm your children with the food they need to have their brain working at maximum power through the day.
- Provide a safe environment for your children and their friends to play actively; encourage swimming, biking, skating, bowling, ball sports, jump rope and other fun activities.
- Eat five to eight small meals a day and keep that metabolism on high.

- Reduce the amount of time spent watching TV. Limit TV watching to weekends and then only two hours per day.
- Eliminate the SUPER SIZE MEAL mentality. Eat smaller portions and teach your children to eat only when they are hungry.
- Eat meals together as a family as often as possible.
- Encourage your children to drink 6–8 glasses of water a day. If you are drinking only bottled water, remember your children are not benefiting from the fluoride in tap water. Fluoride protects their teeth enamel. Consider putting a filter on your sink and drink tap water.
- Stock the refrigerator with low fat foods such as yogurt, fat-free milk, fresh fruit and vegetables. If you don't buy soft drinks, they won't drink them. Don't buy potato chips and Doritos unless you want your children to eat them. HEALTH BEGINS WITH PRUDENT SHOPPING AT THE GROCERY STORE.

Your children will be the only evidence you walked this earth. They are a precious asset; take good care of them.

38. WHAT ARE CARBOHYDRATES AND ARE THEY BAD FOR YOU?

Let your moderation be known unto all men. The Lord [is] at hand.
ڭ Philippians 4:5

Carbohydrates are a food group and as such are a nutrient the body needs. Carbohydrates are commonly known as SUGAR, FIBER AND STARCHES, and come from a wide array of foods—bread, rice, beans, milk, popcorn, potatoes, cookies, spaghetti, corn, and cherry pie. They also come in a variety of forms. The basic building blocks of a carbohydrate are sugar molecules. Starches and fibers are essentially chains of sugar molecules.

There are two main types of carbohydrates: The simple carbohydrates include fruit sugars (fructose), corn and grape sugars (dextrose or glucose) and table sugars (sucrose). Complex carbohydrates include anything with three or more links of sugars. Remember sugar is the main fuel for the body. The brain especially needs it to function, and the brain functions 24 hours a day/ 7 days a week/365 days a year/all the years of your life!

When you eat a carbohydrate, your stomach and digestive system tries to break the carbohydrate down into one sugar molecule, which is then carried into the blood stream and into your cells by insulin. The sugar molecule cannot be used as fuel until it is carried into the cell by insulin. The sugar just sits in the blood and turns into acid—too much sugar in the blood is called diabetes and too much acid in the blood will cause death. Fiber is an exception. It is put together in such a way that it can't be broken down into sugar molecules, and so passes through the body mostly undigested.

So if sugar or carbohydrate is the fuel that the body needs, why do so many experts think carbohydrates are bad? Well, there are many thoughts. The newest one is known as the GYLCEMIC INDEX. This is a new system for classifying carbohydrates and measures how fast and how far blood sugar rises after you eat foods that contains carbohydrates. White bread, for example, is digested almost immediately to glucose, causing blood sugar to spike rapidly. So white bread is classified as having a high glycemic index. Brown rice, in contrast, is digested more slowly, causing a lower and gentler change in blood sugar. It has a lower glycemic index. It is known that the rapid rising and falling in blood sugar damages the inner lining of your blood vessels throughout your body—even the little tiny blood vessels in your heart and brain. Diets filled with high-glycemic-index foods, which cause quick and strong increases in blood sugar levels, have been linked to an increased risk for both diabetes and heart disease. On the other hand, lower glycemic index foods have been shown to help control type 2 diabetes.

One of the most important factors that determines a food's glycemic index is how highly processed its carbohydrates are. Processing carbohydrates removes the fiber-rich outer bran and the vitamin- and mineral-rich inner germ. What's left is mostly the starchy endosperm. Other factors that influence how quickly the carbohydrates in food raise blood sugar include:

- *Fiber content.* Fiber shields the starchy carbohydrates in food from immediate and rapid attack by digestive enzymes. This slows the release of sugar molecules into the bloodstream.
- *Ripeness.* Ripe fruits and vegetables tend to have more sugar than unripe ones, and so tend to have a higher glycemic index.
- *Type of starch.* Starch comes in many different configurations. Some are easier to break into sugar molecules than others. The starch in potatoes, for example, is digested and absorbed into the bloodstream relatively quickly.
- *Fat content and acid content.* The more fat or acid a food contains, the slower its carbohydrates are converted to sugar and absorbed into the bloodstream.
- *Physical form.* Finely ground grain is more rapidly digested, and so has a higher glycemic index, than more coarsely ground grain.

The simple message is to keep processed carbohydrates out of your shopping carts, homes and therefore, diets. Whenever possible, replace highly processed grains, cereals, and sugars with minimally processed whole-grain products. When you are eating at fast food and other restaurants, avoid buying those foods with highly processed carbohydrates. Avoid those snack foods, which contain highly processed carbohydrates.

Be a smart consumer and enjoy all life has to offer!

39. LOW CARB DIETS—A WAY OF LIFE OR A QUICK FIX?

Consider what I say; and the Lord give thee understanding in all things.
                            ᴑᴔ 2 Timothy 2:7

A diet can be defined as the usual food and drink consumed by a person or animal; most Americans, however, understand the concept of a diet as being the act of restricting food intake or the act of restricting the intake of particular foods. Low carbohydrate diets do just that; the "low carb" diets restrict the grams of carbohydrates that should be consumed in a particular day so the body can 1) burn your stores of carbohydrates for fuel and 2) change the rate of metabolism of the carbohydrates you eat and store.

The main way the body stores carbohydrates is in the form of fat. Fat is just a complex form of carbohydrate. When you think about it, if we constantly eat sugars, the body will burn the sugars we eat and not have to burn the sugars that are stored (fat) which is why some diet plans restrict carbohydrates. Fat will be burned for fuel if the body senses that it is out of sugar. The longer it takes to break down a carbohydrate, the longer the dietary carbohydrate you consumed will take to enter the blood stream. While this is happening, your body will have to either 1) burn the stored fat and turn it into sugar or 2) slow down the metabolism to meet the supply of sugar. Many people believe that people who are overweight have two problems: A) people who are overweight slow their metabolism down to the point that it keeps pace with the sugar circulating in the blood stream and B) people who are overweight become very good at changing sugar into fat very quickly.

So what's the answer to the question? Our suggestion is that if you are overweight, instead of searching for diets (low fat, low carb or otherwise) that are quick fixes, you need to incorporate the following lifestyle changes:

- Speed up your metabolism so you can burn more sugars. Any activity will speed up your metabolism if you sustain the activity over 20 minutes and increase your heart rate. Before you try to jog, why not just walk slowly at first, then briskly. This will speed up your metabolism if you do it often and long enough.

- Change the carbohydrates you consume to complex carbohydrates—like whole grains, peas, beans, fresh fruits, and cereals, and fresh vegetables.
- Eat smaller portion sizes—here's a helper hint. Give yourself the serving size you normally do. Your brain is fixed at that level. Count to 60 and then put half back. Do this for a week and then cut the portion size again. It's better to eat ten small meals a day than three large meals that could feed ten people each time.
- Drink 6–8 glasses of water a day.

If you have achieved your ideal and healthy weight and body type, then continue with the tips above!

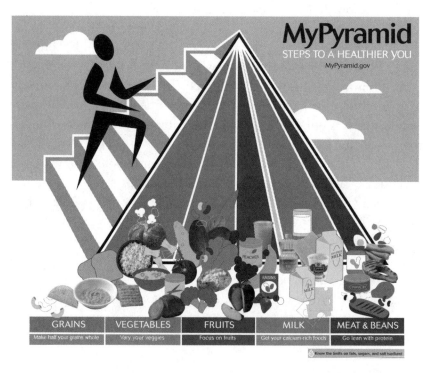

The new 2005 healthy eating food pyramid from the USDA Center for Nutrition Policy and Promotion

40. GENTLEMEN ARE NEVER OBESE

A husband should love his wife as much as Christ loved the Church.

ᐁ Ephesians 5:25

According to the Centers for Disease Control, 61% of adults and 25% of children and adolescents in the United State are overweight. This is primarily due to overeating and to the fact that 40% of us do not engage in leisure physical activities. The dramatic change in overall physique from the past to present can be seen by comparing family photos from the past with photos from today.

Although the media focus has been on the even higher rates of overweight and obesity among African-American women, African-American men also suffer from high rates of excess weight. This excess weight substantially increases the risks of diabetes, stroke, cancer and even arthritis. In fact, obese adults have twice the rate of premature death and disability than the average sized person in the United States. The high rate of obesity among African Americans is unacceptable. African-Americans over seventy years old are not obese. What do you think happened to those who were obese?

Instead of experimenting with fad diets to lose weight and joining health clubs that you never use, doctors currently recommend that you exercise daily and eat a little less. The difference between what an average-sized person and what an obese person consumes is not very much. It turns out that the average obese person eats, or fails to burn up, just 150 excess calories per day. That difference is just about a small bag of potato chips or a can of soda. But it adds up to more that 50,000 extra calories per year that can add ten pounds of fat. Over 20 years, the person who is consuming 150 extra calories per day will have added an extra 200 pounds.

Society encourages us to avoid exertion and become sluggards, to take escalators instead of walking up stairs. Older people, who are quite capable of walking, cannot make their way through an airport without repeated offers to push them in a wheelchair. Even when we try to walk somewhere, someone is always offering to drive us. Golfers cannot walk anymore — carts are required.

A gentleman is never obese for many reasons. First of all, gentlemen never eat in fast-food restaurants — how uncivilized! Other than forgiving others for their transgressions, gentlemen generally do not do things quickly. They like to savor the moment, smell the roses and enjoy God's gifts to us. In addition to regular exercise and a prudent diet, men can easily burn up an extra 150 calories per day performing gentlemanly deeds. Actively greeting others, opening car doors, pulling out chairs, putting on coats, carrying packages, grooming ourselves, keeping our cars, shoes and clothes clean and presentable — all of these little courtesies burn calories. Old men are fond of telling young men to always smile at ladies and find opportunities to be helpful and courteous. They delight in rescuing damsels in distress. You may suspect that they did this to win favor with the ladies only to discover that the true motivation is to look sharp and debonair. A sure sign that you are in the presence of a gentleman is if the lady is obese, because a gentleman does everything for his lady.

SECTION IV

LIVING WITH
HEART DISEASE

41. EARLY WARNING SIGNS OF A HEART ATTACK

For God hath not given us the spirit of fear; but power, and of love, and of a sound mind.

ॐ 2 Timothy 1:7

Every hour, someone in this country dies suddenly from a heart attack. Some of those deaths could have been avoided if the victims or those around them had recognized the early warning signs. By knowing the signs, you can seek help faster and have a much better chance of surviving the heart attack. Speed is especially important because your brain will die if your heart stops for longer than five minutes.

You may be having a heart attack if you experience:

- Dizziness
- Palpitations
- Uncomfortable pressure
- Squeezing
- Pain in the chest lasting more than two minutes.
- Sweating
- Nausea
- Shortness of breath
- Sudden weakness

If you experience any of these symptoms, seek medical help immediately. In most cases, your best first stop is the nearest hospital emergency room. Don't try to drive. Have someone else take you or call 911.

It is normal to deny something as serious as a heart attack could be happening to you. Too often, people who are beginning to have heart attack symptoms tell themselves it is gas, a sore muscle or fatigue. But now that you know the signs, don't take unnecessary chances with your life. Get medical attention at the first sign of heart attack symptoms.

42. WEAR A RED DRESS AND FIGHT HEART DISEASE IN WOMEN (IN FEBRUARY)

And Adam called his wife's name Eve; because she was the mother of all living things.

ᏛᏙ Genesis 3:20

Most women are not aware that heart disease is the number one killer of women. Not breast cancer, cervical cancer, AIDS, or violence—it is heart disease. The "Go Red for Heart Disease" campaign has been launched to make sure women in American know that heart disease kills over 500,000 women each year. The greatest risk for death comes from heart attacks! A heart attack is caused when the muscles of your heart do not get the oxygen and blood supply they need to function because of coronary artery disease. The coronary arteries are responsible for getting blood to the muscles of your heart. If they are clogged or narrowed, the amount of blood going to the muscles of your heart will be reduced. The reasons your coronary arteries will be clogged are because of:

- increased levels of bad cholesterol or low-density lipoprotein.
- uncontrolled blood pressure.
- being overweight.
- uncontrolled stress.
- smoking.
- excessive alcohol.
- lack of exercise.

In general, women can control their risk of developing heart disease by controlling those lifestyle factors which put them at risk for premature death and disability from heart disease. Women are the health care officers for their family. They control what foods are purchased and therefore consumed by our families. Just controlling food consumption will go a long way to limit heart disease by ensuring you are at an optimal weight and your blood pressure and cholesterol are under control. If you smoke, you know you are putting yourself at risk and that goes for excessive alcohol intake and lack of exercise, too.

Join the movement and let's eliminate premature death and disability of women from heart disease. Join the Red Dress campaign — buy a red dress and wear it with pride during heart month (February).

43. WHAT IS CONGESTIVE HEART FAILURE OR DROPSY?

. . . Let us draw near to God with a sincere heart in full assurance of faith, having our hearts sprinkled to cleanse us from a guilty conscience and having our bodies washed with pure water.

ை Hebrews 10:22

Your heart is a pump which has two sides, the right side and left side. The veins in your body bring back blood which has waste and low oxygen. This blood comes to the right side of the heart and the right side of the heart pumps this "bad" blood to the lungs, which blow off the waste (carbon dioxide) and replaces it with oxygen. This good blood (oxygen-rich blood) goes to the left side of the heart where it pumps the good blood back to the body through the aorta.

Heart failure is a condition in which the heart can't act as an efficient pump to pump the oxygen-rich blood from the lungs to the rest of the body. When this happens, the blood backs up to the lungs and eventually to the right side of the heart, which will take the blood back to the venous system. When the blood backs up to the lungs, you have fluid on the lungs which makes it hard to breathe. Our lungs need air to get oxygen; humans do not have gills like fish and therefore we cannot extract oxygen from water. When the lungs fill up with blood, which contains water, we cannot breathe, which is why if you have heart failure you will feel anxious because your body cannot get the oxygen it needs.

Your heart pump can break down for many reasons. One of the most common reasons your heart pump breaks down is because you have had a *heart attack*. When you have a heart attack it can damage the muscles of the heart which means the heart can't function normally as a pump. Other things that can damage the heart and cause the heart to have pump failure are as follows:

- **High Blood Pressure**. If the left side of the heart has to pump against higher and higher blood pressures, it will make the heart muscle weak.
- **Heart Valve Disease Due to Past Rheumatic Fever or Other Causes.** If your heart valves don't close properly, the chambers of your heart become bigger and don't function as well as it should.
- **Primary Disease of The Heart Muscle Itself, Called Cardiomyopathy.** The muscles of the heart get attacked by bacteria or viruses and become weak. This will weaker the heart muscles and cause the heart pump to fail. Remember the lady who Bette Midler sang the song to in the movie *Beaches*? She died from viral cardiomyopathy!
- **Heart Defects Present At Birth—Congenital Heart Defects.** This can either be a valve problem, a heart pump problem, or both.

Your failing heart will keep on working but because it can't pump blood normally, the fluid will back up to your lungs or to your legs. The swelling of the legs is commonly referred to as **dropsy** or **edema**. When you have heart failure, your other organs don't get the blood supply they need and you might get kidney failure and liver failure. Heart failure is no fun to have, therefore you need to make sure you do the things necessary to prevent it - like get your blood pressure under control, stop smoking, and lose weight.

The good news is that heart failure can be treated. Your doctor can prescribe medications that will help you treat heart failure. There are things you can do to help the medicine work better, like:

- getting the proper rest
- eating food low in salt
- modify daily activities
- drugs such as
  - ACE (angiotensin-converting enzyme) inhibitors
  - beta blockers
  - digitalis

- water pills (diuretics)
- vasodilators
- pills with nitrates

Various drugs are used in combination to treat congestive heart failure. Ask you doctor for the best combination for you. Also, if you are an African American with heart failure there are exciting, new drugs for you as well that contain nitrous oxide. Ask your doctor about them.

When a specific cause of congestive heart failure is discovered, it should be treated or, if possible, corrected. For example, some cases of heart failure can be treated by treating high blood pressure. If the heart failure is caused by an abnormal heart valve, the valve can be surgically replaced.

If the heart becomes so damaged that it can't be repaired, a more drastic approach should be considered. A pacemaker or a heart transplant could be options.

Most people with mild and moderate heart failure can be treated. Proper medical supervision can prevent them from becoming incapacitated.

Remember, you only have one heart; take good care of it.

44. STROKE

But be ye doers of the word, and not hearers only, deceiving your own selves.

ᏀᎯ James 1:22

Some facts about stroke:

- Stroke is the third leading cause of death in the United States.
- 500,000 new strokes occur each year.
- Hypertension, diabetes, cigarette smoking, heart rhythm irregularities and high blood cholesterol are major risk factors.

Recognize the early warning signs of stroke. Work with your doctor a good prevention program, including diet and exercise. Early warning signs of stroke include:

- Numbness or drooping of the face
- Weakness of the arm or leg especially on the same side of the body
- Sudden severe, unexplained headache
- Sudden blurred vision
- Unexplained dizziness or falls, especially along with the other symptoms

  Remember, most strokes are not painful.

If you have any of these "Warning Signs" don't wait! Every second counts in stopping the damage caused by stroke. Call 911.

Controlling your blood pressure can protect you against stroke. Prompt and appropriate treatment will save your life.

45. HARDENING OF THE ARTERIES

And when they came out of the boat, immediately the people recognized Him, ran through that whole surrounding region, and began to carry about on beds those who were sick to wherever they heard He was. Wherever He entered, into villages, cities, or the country, they laid the sick in the marketplace, and begged Him that they might just touch the border of His garment. And as many as touched Him were made well.

ᘒ Mark 6:54–56

Atherosclerosis describes what happens when your arteries become narrowed with plaque: your blood can't freely get through the arteries to feed the cells which make up your body.

Plaque is made up of calcium deposits, cholesterol, and dead cells. Pieces of plaque can break off and start flowing with the blood, and clog up smaller arteries downstream. Eventually, this condition may cause strokes, heart attacks, or kidney failure, and can also seriously weaken the blood flow to the legs.

You can prevent atherosclerosis by:

- Controlling your weight and blood pressure
- Not smoking
- Cutting back on animal fats in your diet
- Exercising for at least thirty minutes every day

Here are some common treatments for atherosclerosis:

- *Balloon angioplasty.* In this procedure, a surgeon inserts an uninflated balloon into the clogged artery, and, by blowing it up, squeezes the plaque to the sides of the artery, creating a larger channel for the blood to pass through.
- *Coronary artery bypass* creates new plumbing, using veins from the leg to direct blood past the clogged arteries in the heart.
- *Laser surgery* burns up whatever is blocking the arteries
- What we can call rotor-rooter system of surgery which lets the surgeon do the same thing a plumber would do with a clogged drain.

Treating atherosclerosis is far better than not treating it. But best of all, avoid it. You can help yourself out by crossing the following items out of your diet:

- Cigarette smoking
- Hamburgers
- Sausages
- Pizza
- Hot dogs
- Doughnuts

Just taking these simple steps will greatly improve your health and your chances of living a long life. You can also help keep athero-sclerosis under control by exercising regularly, and eating more fruits, vegetables, whole grains, and cereals.

46. PERFORM A DEATH-DEFYING ACT: GET YOUR BLOOD PRESSURE UNDER CONTROL

And these words which I command thee this day, shall be in thine heart.
ᖇ Deuteronomy 6:6

The term *high blood pressure* came into common usage about thirty years ago when researchers began to recognize it as the number one killer of Americans. High blood pressure, because it has no symptoms, is a silent thief that steals someone's friend or relative every minute of every day.

To understand high blood pressure, you need to know that all the cells in our bodies need blood rich in oxygen and other nutrients in order to do their work. This enriched blood helps us to move muscles, to taste, to feel, and to stay alive.

As the body consumes energy, it also creates waste, so the body needs a way to remove this garbage. Picking up the garbage that the cells produce is another job of the heart and the blood vessels (the cardiovascular system). Feeding the cells and removing waste is a big job. To do it, the heart pumps 100,000 times per day, every day we live.

For reasons we don't fully understand, in one of four Americans, the pressure that pushes blood around the body increases beyond safe limits. If you keep up the pressure on anything, something has to give. In the case of high blood pressure, what usually gives are the vessels that deliver blood to your brain, kidneys, and heart, resulting in stroke, kidney failure, congestive heart failure, and heart attack.

Blood pressure is reported in two numbers. The higher number describes the pressure in the blood vessels when the heart is at work pushing the blood out. This is called the *systolic*. The lower number, the *diastolic*, describes the heart at rest, being filled up with blood. The safe limit for blood pressure is less than or equal to 140/90mm Hg. Numbers above this limit usually require treatment with medicine to reduce the risk of a stroke or heart attack. In general, the lower the number, the lower the risk.

To avoid the consequences of high blood pressure, get your blood pressure checked. If it is too high, see a doctor about it. If you are placed on treatment, follow the doctor's advice, not just for a while but for the rest of your life. Develop a partnership with your doctor to ensure your continued good health.

High blood pressure is one high you do not want. Perform a death-defying act and get your blood pressure under control.

47. CONTROLLING YOUR BLOOD PRESSURE

Then they cried out to the Lord in their trouble. And He saved them out of their distresses. He sent His word and healed them, And delivered them from their destructions.

❧ Psalm 107:19,20

Pressure in our arteries is necessary to keep the blood circulating. But when the pressure is too high, there is greater risk that weak sections of our blood vessels will rupture, or that the inside of the blood vessels will become rough, causing clots to develop. The increased pressure also causes the heart to work harder, become larger, weaker (heart failure), and eventually just give out.

People who have high blood pressure are at greater risk of stroke, heart attack, congestive heart failure, kidney failure, and blindness. The higher the blood pressure, the greater the risk.

The good news is that high blood pressure is easily detected and easily controlled. So get your blood pressure checked. The test is simple, and it may lead to a longer life.

If you have been diagnosed with high blood pressure:

- Maintain your ideal weight. If you are overweight, for every three pounds you lose, your blood pressure will go down two millimeters. Every little bit helps.
- Increase the amount of exercise you do, but follow your doctor's advice about how much exercise is good for you.
- Reduce the amount of salt in your diet.
- Keep your appointments with your doctor.
- Take medication as prescribed by your doctor. Establish a routine for when and where you will take your medication.
- Check your blood pressure regularly. You may want to do this at home with a device you can purchase at a drug store. Ask your doctor about this.

- If you take blood pressure medicine and experience side effects (such as drowsiness, constipation, coughing or headaches) don't stop your medication, but tell your doctor about the side effects so adjustments can be made.
- Do not take any prescription medication not prescribed for you, and do not give yours to anyone else.
- Tell your doctor all the medications you are taking, including over-the-counter medications, such as aspirin.
- Be sure you understand when to take your medication — whether before meals, after meals, on an empty stomach, or before bed.

48. CHILDREN AND HEART DISEASE

We are God's offspring, for in Him we live and move and have our being.
ᕲ Acts 17:28

In general, heart disease affects older people. It's also true that children can handle more junk food than adults without immediate health consequences. But this doesn't mean there are no long-term consequences. The dietary habits of a lifetime begin in childhood, and, for that reason, heart disease starts in childhood, too.

Autopsy studies done on American soldiers killed in Korea and Vietnam showed advanced clogging in their arteries. Most of these soldiers were in their teens and early twenties. Their condition resulted from a diet of doughnuts, sodas, hamburgers, steaks, ribs, hot dogs, sausages, and other animal products. On the other hand, autopsies of Korean soldiers who ate mostly vegetables and rice revealed no buildup of plaque or blockage in their arteries. Studies by Dr. Gerald Berenson show that American children, Black and White, of both sexes had elevated cholesterol and blocking of arteries even at ten years old.

The best time to get children to eat right and exercise regularly is early. If your children test high for cholesterol, do not panic! You just have to be more conscientious about what they eat. When Guatemalan children were taken off their high vegetable diet and placed on an American diet, they developed elevated cholesterol after just one month. (Do you realize that the filling in Twinkies is made with sugar and lard?) But you can reverse the process just as quickly, by getting your children off Twinkies and other fast foods and prepared foods that can endanger their health.

You talk to your children about not getting into a stranger's car and about looking both ways before crossing the street. It is also time you talk to them about eating a balanced diet that is low in fats and sugar. Remind them that besides letting them live longer, healthier lives, such a diet will also help their athletic performance and their good looks. That way you appeal to both their intelligence and their sense of self.

Let children of both sexes go shopping with you so you can teach them how to read food labels. Let them cook with you so you can teach them how to discard the skin from chicken, to use olive oil instead of lard or palm oil, and to refrigerate soup and sauces so the fat can be skimmed off.

Most important, get them to snack on vegetables, pretzels and fruits instead of Twinkies, candy bars, donuts, potato chips and cakes. Help them to establish a healthy lifestyle. Good eating is healthy, and it also can be fun!

---

49. LIVING WITH DIABETES

Let the word of Christ dwell in you richly in all wisdom; teaching and admonishing one another in psalms and hymns and spiritual songs, singing with grace in your hearts to the Lord.

ᕫ Colossians 3:16

All the cells of the body, and especially the brain cells, need sugar to function properly. The blood releases sugar to the cells when the cells are stimulated by insulin, a hormone produced by the pancreas.

When your body does not make enough insulin or you're loading up on sugar heavier than your insulin can keep up with it, you develop diabetes.

All types of diabetes (diabetes mellitus, hyperglycemia, or just plain diabetes) occur when the body can't properly store and use blood sugar, also called *glucose*.

One-out-of-four Americans who have diabetes don't know they have it, so recognize the signs. You may have diabetes if:

- You are excessively thirsty.
- You urinate frequently.
- You get overly tired for no apparent reason.
- Someone in your family has a history of diabetes.
- You are overweight.
- You have bruises, cuts or infections that just do not heal, and/or you often have an itch.

The more overweight and the older you are, the more likely you are to have this condition.

Diabetes is easy to detect and control, but if you overlook or neglect it, serious consequences, like blindness, sores that will not heal, kidney failure, coma, and stroke, can follow. Treated properly, diabetics continue to feel well and live like anyone else.

Many people control diabetes by taking oral medications. Others require daily injections of insulin. Although insulin treatment is not a cure, conscientious patients can live normal lives with it. Daily injections can supply the missing hormone, though they can't make the pancreas work again.

Besides medication and regular examinations by your doctor, weight management, diet, and exercise are the three best ways to control diabetes. If you are overweight, lose weight. Losing ten pounds will make a big difference by reducing your need for insulin. Exercise is important because besides helping you keep both your weight and stress down, it helps keep many parts of your body, including your heart and lungs, healthy.

50. AN ASPIRIN A DAY KEEPS THE GRIM REAPER AWAY

For we walk by faith, not by sight.

⧉ 1 Corinthians 5: 7

Most of us keep a very important medicine in our pocket books, medicine cabinets or on the kitchen counter. The medicine is Aspirin. This drug is widely available, very cheap and doesn't require a prescription from your doctor. It can save your life if you are having a heart attack.

The symptoms of a heart attack are:

- Dizziness
- Palpitations
- Uncomfortable pressure
- Squeezing
- Pain in the center of the chest
- Sweating
- Nausea
- Shortness of breath
- Sudden weakness

These symptoms by themselves may not signal a heart attack. However in combination, they could definitely be a life-threatening emergency. The Association of Black Cardiologists recommends that anyone having symptoms of a heart attack, call 911 and chew a 325 mg tablet (1 adult Aspirin) of Aspirin.

Aspirin is also effective in lowering your risk of developing a stroke. Most adults who take one low dose aspirin a day also cut their risk of having a stroke by one-half or 50 percent. When you have your first glass of water in the morning also take 81mgs of aspirin.

Taking a daily low dose daily aspirin is no substitute for living the kind of life that promotes good cardiovascular health. Getting to your ideal weight and ideal body mass index (BMI), exercising and limiting your stress are better than taking that buffered Aspirin. However, if you think you are at increased risk for having a stroke, talk to your doctor and find out if it's okay for you to take an Aspirin a day or every other day. Your doctor will know if there are any reasons for you not to take Aspirin, especially if you are on a blood thinner or have a bleeding ulcer. So check in with your doctor to see if it's okay for you to keep the Grim Reaper Away with an Aspirin a DAY.

51. DO I NEED A BLOOD THINNER?

That thou mightest know the certainty of those things, wherein thou hast been instructed.

ꙮ Luke 1:4

Your doctor may prescribe a blood thinner if you have had a heart valve replaced or if you have medical conditions such as atrial fibrillation, phlebitis (blood clots in your veins), congestive heart failure, or, in some cases, if you are obese. Blood thinners or anticoagulants reduce your risk for heart attack, stroke, and blockages in your arteries and veins by preventing clumps of blood (blood clots) from forming or growing. However, blood thinners cannot break up blood clots which have already formed.

How do blood thinners work?

Blood thinners are part of a class of medicines called anticoagulants. Although they are called blood thinners, these medicines do not really thin your blood. Instead, they decrease the blood's ability to clot. Decreased clotting keeps fewer harmful blood clots from forming and from blocking blood vessels.

Oral anticoagulants can come in a pill form that you swallow or can be given to you through your veins. The blood thinners that are given to you through your veins are more powerful; these blood thinners are given to you by your doctor when you are at immediate risk for developing a stroke or heart attack. If you are given this more powerful blood thinner in the hospital, the doctor will send you home on the blood thinner you take in pill form. The pill is called Coumadin and the blood thinner given to you through your veins is called Heparin.

Other medicines you may be taking can increase or decrease the effect of blood thinners. Be sure to tell your doctor about every medicine and vitamin or herbal supplement you are taking, so he or she can tell you about any interactions.

The following are categories of medicines that can increase or decrease the effects of blood thinners. Because there are so many kinds of medicines within each category, not every type of medicine is listed by name. Tell your doctor about every medicine you are taking, even if it is not listed below.

- Aspirin
- Acetaminophen (e.g., Tylenol, Excedrin)
- Ibuprofen (e.g., Motrin, Advil, Nuprin)
- Ketoprofen (e.g., Orudis, Orudis KT)
- Naproxen (e.g., Aleve)
- Medicines to treat an irregular heartbeat (antiarrhythmics)
- Antacids
- Corticosteroids or other cortisone-like medicines
- Antidepressants
- Antihistamines
- Calcium and vitamin K supplements
- Sleeping pills
- Certain antibiotics
- Certain medicines used to treat convulsions
- Medicines used to treat an overactive thyroid
- Certain antifungal medicines

Also, when you are on a blood thinner, you will have to have your blood checked to make sure your blood is not becoming too thin. Make sure you get your blood tested when your doctor asks you to and make sure you understand the results of your test. Your body still needs to clot your blood even if you are on a blood thinner; your doctor is the best person to help you and your body do just that!

SECTION V

PRACTICAL GUIDANCE FOR WOMEN, PREGNANT MOMS AND NEW MOMS

52. BIRTH CONTROL—FACTS AND MYTHS

So God created man in His [own] image, in the image of God created He him; male and female created He them.

             ❧ Genesis 1:27

Having a child is one of the most important decisions a man and a woman will make. Initially, pregnancy commits a woman to 40 weeks of having to care for not only herself, but also the baby she is carrying. After the birth, it commits the parents of this baby to at least 18 years of planning, sharing their lives and altering their lives to include a new human being. Pregnancy should be an active decision that two people make and shouldn't just be the result of having unprotected sex. However, if you are engaging in unprotected sex you are exposing yourself to the possibility of pregnancy, as well as sexually transmitted diseases.

Eighty-five percent of women who use no contraceptives during intercourse become pregnant each year. *The only guarantee against pregnancy is not having vaginal intercourse or to become sterile.*

Other contraceptive methods can *greatly reduce the risk* of pregnancy during intercourse but do not guarantee you will not get pregnant. If you have made the decision to engage in sex and do not want to be pregnant, the choice of which contraception you choose can varying depending on your needs, and may change throughout your life. To decide which method to use now, you need to know:

- How well will it fit into your lifestyle?
- How convenient will it be?
- How effective will it be?
- How safe will it be?
- How affordable will it be?
- How reversible will it be?
- Will it protect against sexually transmitted diseases?

Some women choose the behavioral methods to contraception such as continuous abstinence, the withdrawal method, outercourse or continuous breast-feeding. Of the four behavioral methods, only abstinence can guarantee 100 percent contraception.

Some women choose the hormone method. The most commonly used hormone is progestin alone or in combination with estrogens. Both hormones occur naturally in a women's body and when given in a pill form will either fool the body not to release an egg or change the uterus not to accept the egg. With the hormone methods, especially low dose hormones, unless the woman is taking the pills exactly as prescribed, an egg can get released or implanted. Every time an egg gets released it can get fertilized during vaginal intercourse and then be implanted in the uterus, thus producing a pregnancy.

Some examples of the hormone method are implants, a patch, a shot that lasts three months and the pill. Women should pick which method or hormone therapy works best for them and talk with their doctor before taking hormones.

Women can also use barrier devices such as a vaginal condom or diaphragm. The woman can also request her partner also use a condom. The barrier methods are not foolproof and if the woman is ovulating the sperm from the male can get to the egg and fertilize it. If you are going to use the barrier method, it is advised that you combine it with a spermicidal cream to decrease the chance that a live sperm will make it to the egg and fertilize it.

Another form of birth control is an implantable device that is inserted into the uterus–the IUD. This works by preventing a fertilized egg from implanting in the uterus. Most fertilized eggs implant at a certain spot in the uterus which is where the IUD is placed. There are many "IUD" babies. This means fertilized eggs often find other places in the uterus to implant itself and grow.

Another form of birth control is sterilization. A woman can have her tubes tied, have her uterus removed or both. A man can also get his tubes tied. Sterilization is a permanent form of birth control and before a woman or man engages in this choice they should be clear that having children is not an option. You can get your tubes untied.

However, the chances of pregnancy is lowered even when the man's or the women's tube are untied because of scar tissue in the tubes and in men, antibodies develop to the sperm and make them less potent. The choice of sterilization is an important one and should be discussed thoroughly.

The choices of available birth control are many and neither the man nor the woman should rely on their partner to protect against pregnancy. Since the woman has to carry the pregnancy, the woman should at least be sure she has taken the precautions she needs not to conceive if that is her choice. The man should also realize that each vaginal intercourse could lead to pregnancy unless he is sure his sperm is not going to fertilize an egg. Both partners should know that unless condoms are used, neither is protected against sexually transmitted diseases.

If you are mature enough to have sex, be mature enough to protect yourself from unwanted pregnancies and unwanted sexually transmitted diseases.

53. SPARE THE ROD AND SPOIL THE CHILD

Provoke not your children to wrath lest they be discouraged.

ҩ Colossians 3:21

Disciplining children just got harder, because it is no longer acceptable to "hit them upside their head", beat them with a switch, or shake them the old-fashioned way. Children will forever be children and boys will be boys, so their behavior still needs to be corrected so they can succeed in modern society.

Experts disagree on what "good discipline" means today. But there is some basic agreement in their thinking. Children need boundaries because they don't know how to set boundaries themselves. They learn from their parents. So, if they have parents who cannot set boundaries, children grow up with the idea that boundaries are not necessary, even though we live in a society where they will be severely punished if they don't respect boundaries.

A child's natural inclination is "I want what I want, when I want it," whether it's good for them or not. God provided children with parents to teach them right from wrong. Most children respond to specific rules and regulations, and to guidance as to the difference between right and wrong. On occasion, children specifically disobey their parents. The challenge to parents is to communicate their authority and their need to be obeyed. Here are some helpful guidelines for discipline that you may want to keep in mind:

- *That which is followed by something pleasurable is likely to be repeated. That which is followed by something unpleasant is likely not to be repeated.* Make specific note of the behaviors you want to decrease and use methods the child doesn't like. This can include turning your back on them or not speaking to them. Also make specific note of behaviors you want, including doing their homework and responding politely. Smiles, hugs and kisses, even more than money, TV privileges and a "treat", are excellent ways to reinforce the positive behaviors you want to see in your child.

- *Reinforce authority*: Children have to learn to respect all adults and not just their parents. This behavior is essential if the child is to succeed in school. Children should be taught at an early age that adults should be listened to and they are not equals with adults. A good technique is to train your children to say "Yes, ma'am" or "No, sir." Understanding authority is an essential part of success in our society.
- *Keep a cool head*: When disciplining your children, you have to remain in control. Otherwise, the child sees you out of control and decides his or her transgression isn't the issue. You can't trust your judgment when you're angry. Anger leads to impulsive actions and poor problem-solving skills. If you find yourself seeing red, take a time out for yourself. Count to ten (or fifty), and take some good, deep breaths before you act. If you make the mistake of hitting your child just because you are tired and frustrated, the problem will get worse.
- *Be consistent*: Easier said than done. It is important, though, to enforce your rules consistently. Otherwise, children get a mixed message about whether their behavior is acceptable or not.
- *Be timely*: It's much more effective to respond to a negative behavior immediately after it occurs, rather than use the "wait until your father gets home" response. Denying a child dessert in the evening for misbehavior in the morning is not effective. Children are spatially-oriented human beings—they can't connect the dots in the abstract so the punishment has to match the crime and has to be immediate. DO something at the moment to show the child that his or her behavior has consequences.
- *Use age-appropriate strategies*: Your discipline strategies will and should differ, depending on the age of the child. For example, when an 8 month old starts tearing books or chewing on shoes, you can use a technique of **remove and distract**. Time outs can be used with toddlers. A timeout is literally meant to

be "time out from positive reinforcement." That means you select a timeout area that is rather boring (not their room full of toys). Time-out should not be done in closets or any place frightening or dangerous for the child.

- *Use repetition and patience:* Discipline doesn't just mean discouraging problem behaviors. It means encouraging and enforcing appropriate behavior. As soon as children learn to talk, we should expect them to say "please" and "thank-you".
- *Solicit help from grandparents, uncles, aunts, ministers and other people the child respects:* Gang-up and use group pressure to produce desirable behaviors.

If you follow the helpful hints above there should be no need for spankings. Excessive punishment is not good because children become defensive and just tune out parents. Whatever discipline you use, make sure it matches the transgression, the temperament and age of your child.

54. CONGRATULATIONS! YOU'RE HAVING A BABY!

Children, obey your parents in the Lord, for this is right. Honor thy father and mother; which is the first commandment with a promise.

ᑌ Ephesians 6:1–2

Having a baby is one of life's greatest pleasures, but it's also a time when a lot will be required of both Mom and Dad, during the pregnancy and after. The most important ingredient in having a healthy baby is a healthy Mom. Healthy Mom, healthy baby. Happy Mom, happy baby. The baby will be exposed to everything the Mom exposes herself to, so it is important that pregnant Moms get as healthy as possible before their pregnancy and maintain an optimal state of health during and after the pregnancy. Here's why it is so important for Moms to be healthy when pregnant:

- The baby's environment for 40 weeks is within the Mom's uterus, so if the Mom smokes, the baby smokes. Smoking is not good for mature, adult lungs and is definitely not good for young, developing lungs.
- If the Mom exposes herself to recreational drugs and alcohol, the baby is exposed to the same things, which are definitely not good for developing hearts, brains and other important organs.
- If the Mom is under stress then the baby will be exposed to stress, which is definitely not good for a developing brain and nervous system.

Babies exposed to unhealthy substances and stress are more likely to leave the womb early and be born prematurely. If a baby is born prematurely, the baby will have low birth weight. Low birth weight babies and premature babies do not develop as normally as babies born at full term and at a normal birth weight. Moms who overeat during their pregnancy put themselves at risk for developing diabetes, and also for making their babies large and prone to being overweight for the rest of their lives.

If the Mom eats healthy, exercises and surrounds herself with a stress-free environment that is full of life and caring, the baby will benefit as well. Babies who are read to or who have songs sung to them are more likely to reach developmental milestones, like walking and talking, at early ages. Babies born to healthy Moms are more likely to engage with other people and form those necessary bonds with the people in their environment.

If you decide to become a Mom, we suggest you plan for your pregnancy to ensure that your environment and the environment for your baby is the best it can be. Here are some helpful hints:

- Pick an OB/GYN physician and make an appointment before you become pregnant. You will have to visit this doctor frequently during your pregnancy, and it's important that you and your doctor are comfortable with each other so that you have effective and optimal communication.
- Have your first pre-natal visit within the first three months of your pregnancy, so that your doctor can ensure that you and the baby are all right.
- During the first six months of your pregnancy, you will usually see your doctor once a month; the visits will become more frequent during your last month of pregnancy.
- During your pregnancy, you should have at least two ultrasounds to make sure that you and your doctor know how many babies you are carrying and that the baby, or babies, are developing normally.
- Be sure to eat healthy foods from the five food groups, and do not gain too much weight. If you think about it, the average baby weights 7 $1/2$ pounds at birth. You have another 10–15 pounds for the amniotic fluid and placenta, so the average woman should only gain about 17–22 pounds during her pregnancy. Pregnancy is not an excuse to overeat!
- If you begin to retain a lot of fluid in your ankles or are having headaches, be sure to call your doctor.
- If there are signs of infection, let your doctor know. Infections, such as urinary tract infections, can cause the baby to come early.

- Get information on breast-feeding. Remember your breast milk is the best form of nourishment your baby can eat.
- Be sure to get plenty of exercise during your pregnancy. Walking helps your pelvic muscles stay loose, which will help you during your labor and delivery.
- Choose a pediatrician and visit the pediatrician during your pregnancy before the baby comes so that you know what visits will be required right after birth. In general, you should take the baby to see the pediatrician within two weeks of going home from the hospital, then at 1 month, two months, four months, six months, nine months, 12 months, 15 months, 18 months, and two yrs. Then at three years and once between the ages of 4–6 years old.

Congratulations! You're having a baby and a wonderful experience awaits you.

55. BREAST FEEDING: WHAT EVERY MOTHER SHOULD KNOW!

So don't be anxious about tomorrow. God will take care of you tomorrow too! Live one day at a time.

k Matthew 6:34

God has a way of giving every one of us what we need to be healthy, wealthy and wise. So much so, that in anticipation of child-bearing, He gave every woman two breasts from which comes the best food your baby can have.

Human milk is healthier for all babies than formula. It is especially healthy for babies that are born prematurely or with low birth weights. Human milk is better for babies for lots of reasons. Here are some:

- Breast milk has helpful antibodies that help children fight disease.
- Breast milk contains immune cells that fight diseases that invade the body through the stomach and intestines.
- Breast fed babies have lower rates for hospital admissions, ear infections, diarrhea, rashes, allergies and other infections.
- Breast milk promotes development in babies.
- Breast milk helps the Mom and baby bond and provides a nurturing environment.
- Breast milk also helps babies prevent dental cavities because the baby isn't left sleeping with a milk bottle in their mouth.

A lot more mothers breast-feed at birth and continue to breast-feed for six months. Actually breast-feeding your child to his or her first birthday is recommended. Even if Moms go back to work six weeks after having their baby, they can breast-feed before and after work and provide breast milk for the baby by pumping their breast and storing the milk to be fed to the baby later. You can add solid foods to the babies diet at four—six months even when breast-feeding. No baby should have cow's milk until their first birthday.

What mothers need to remember is that whatever they eat or drink will show up in their breast milk so if a Mom is going to breast feed she just needs to know what foods she can and cannot eat. Also, every Mom that breast-feeds should drink lots of water, which will make the milk come in faster at the beginning and keep the milk flowing. Some foods may be okay to eat but may give your baby gas or colic. Sometimes it's not clear why a baby develops gas or colic but it's okay because your diet can be adjusted and it will cut down on the amount of gas your baby experiences.

Moms on medication can also breast-feed. Check with your doctor to see what medications can safely be taken while you breast-feed your baby.

Here are some tips for a breast-feeding Mom:

- Start nursing your baby within the first hour of delivery. This will help your milk come in and the early milk, colostrum, contains helpful antibodies for your baby.
- Make sure your nipple is as far back in the baby's mouth as possible.
- Nurse on demand. Don't wake your baby up before your baby is ready, however, most breast-fed babies will want to eat every two to three hours.
- Babies don't need between-meal snacks like sugar water or formula. Your breast milk has all the nutrients and fluids the baby needs.
- Try not to give your baby a pacifier. The sucking required for breast-feeding is different than for pacifiers and may confuse the baby. When babies cry it's usually for a good reason that should be investigated rather than soothed with a pacifier.
- Air-dry your nipples after each feeding to make them strong. If your nipples crack you can put a little vitamin E on them—it won't hurt the baby.
- Your breasts will be full but shouldn't be warm or have painful lumps. If your breasts develop painful lumps or you get a fever you might have an infection and you should call your doctor.
- The last tip may be the most important. In order to produce milk, Moms have to be sure to have plenty of rest, little stress,

6–8 glasses of water a day and eat a health balanced diet. The average Mom only needs to consume an extra 500 calories a day to produce enough milk for her baby, so eat right but not too much!

Above all, enjoy this time with your baby. Baby therapy is good stuff. Time passes quickly and the memories of this first year of life with your baby will satisfy you for the rest of your life.

56. BREAST FIBROIDS—WHAT ARE THEY AND IF I HAVE THEM, WHAT SHOULD I DO?

So God created man in his own image, in the image of God he created him; male and female he created them.

ᴥ Genesis 1:27

Up to 40 percent of American women 35 and older have fibroids. Breast fibroids are moveable, rubbery nodules, which can cause swelling near the breast surface. It is thought that women with excessive amounts of estrogen or an under active thyroid gland will be more prone to fibroids in the breast. Fibroids are not cancer; but any woman with breast fibroids should be evaluated by their doctor, who will more often than not, order a mammogram. Breast fibroids also get bigger depending on your diet. Foods high in fat, caffeine or chocolate can make your breast fibroids grow.

Women with breast fibroids usually have the following symptoms:

- a bumpy, cobblestone feel to the breast
- breasts feeling full
- tenderness and swelling of breasts right before your cycle; this discomfort usually goes away after the cycle
- itching of the nipples

Women should do breast self-exams on a monthly basis; this is especially true of women with breast fibroids. Most women discover their breast cancer long before a mammogram because you can feel an abnormality before it can be detected by the mammogram. To do a breast self test:

- lie on your back and put one arm under your head.
- use your other hand, the second and third fingers, to rub your breast against your chest wall. You should start at the outer rim of the breast and work toward the nipple to massage and feel

your breasts in pie-shaped areas just like the slices of a pizza. Make sure you massage your entire breast.

- The breast tissue should feel lumpy. If you ever feel anything hard immediately seek advice from your doctor.
- Repeat this process with your other breast.

Only about one percent of women with breast fibroids ever develop cancer. Breast cancer can be treated very well if caught early, which is why it is so important for you to do your own breast examinations. Don't act like an ostrich with your head in the sand; do monthly breast exams and be in control of your own life and health.

57. UTERINE FIBROIDS—WHAT ARE THEY AND IF I HAVE THEM WHAT SHOULD I DO?

God blessed them and said to them, "Be fruitful and increase in number; fill the earth and subdue it. Rule over the fish of the sea and the birds of the air and over every living creature that moves on the ground.

∽ Genesis 1: 28

Twenty-five percent of American woman have fibroids in their uterus. You can have just one or many. Many women have them and have no symptoms, but depending on their location and size, woman can have pain or excessive bleeding with their cycles or bleeding in-between cycles.

Fibroids are benign growths in the uterus. For the majority of woman they don't cause a problem and most women don't know they have them. They are usually found on a routine annual exam at which point your physician will watch them. Fibroids are more common in woman of childbearing age, especially in women between the ages of 30 and 40. You may be at greater risk of developing uterine fibroids if you are:

- An African-American woman. African-American women are 3–5 times more likely to have fibroids than white woman.
- Overweight.
- Never been pregnant.

If your fibroids are causing symptoms, the treatment will depend on which symptoms you are having. If you are bleeding a lot, your doctor can prescribe hormones that can shrink your fibroids. If the hormones don't work and you keep bleeding you may have to have your fibroids removed or your uterus removed. Remember, even if you have to have your uterus removed (hysterectomy), ask your doctor to leave your ovaries so that you can continue to secrete female hormones that protect your bones and that prevent you from having hot flashes.

The other reason to have your fibroids removed may be because they are so large that they compress your bladder and make it difficult for you to hold your urine. Another common problem for women with large fibroids is persistent backaches.

Women with fibroids should watch how much caffeine and chocolate they eat. They make the fibroids grow. Stress also makes fibroids grow. Talk with your doctor thoroughly about your fibroids and make careful decisions before you decide to have surgery. Surgery may be the best option but it is certainly not the only one.

58. TAKE A BITE OUT OF TOOTH DECAY

We are "the sweet fragrance of Christ."

❧ 2 Corinthians 2:15

Wouldn't it be wonderful if, for the rest of your life, you never had a cavity or a toothache, and never had gingivitis (gum inflammation) or lost a tooth? That can come true if you follow a few simple rules.

In a nutshell, brush and floss your teeth two times per day, and see your dentist twice a year.

Teeth decay can cause toothaches when sugars from the food you eat react with the bacteria in your mouth to form an acid. That acid eats away at the enamel on the teeth and causes decay.

Many communities have met this problem by adding fluoride to the water. Fluorine hardens teeth and makes them more resistant to decay. But there are also many things you can do for yourself.

Here are ten tips for keeping your teeth strong:

- Brush your teeth after each meal. Take care to brush the gums as well as the backs and tops of the teeth. (If you prefer, you can massage the gums with a clean finger.) You may even want to lightly brush your tongue and the soft parts of your mouth.
- Floss your teeth every day. Flossing gets at the plaque that your toothbrush can't reach. Flossing is simple: insert a piece of dental floss between each of the teeth, especially the back ones, and work the floss back and forth against each tooth to remove food particles that promote gum disease.
- Maintain a good diet with sufficient calcium.
- Get semi-annual dental check-up and cleaning.
- Avoid foods, like sweets, that contain refined sugar.
- Learn to recognize and treat gum disease quickly. (Gum disease is a major cause of tooth loss).

- Don't grind your teeth.
- Don't smoke or chew tobacco.
- Don't use your teeth to remove caps from bottles.
- Start your children off right—take them to a dentist before they are five years old, teach them how to brush and floss, and insist on it. You will have to remind them for about five years, but eventually they will develop the routine. The investment will save them pain and suffering, and save you money later.

59. DOES YOUR BABY NEED A CIRCUMCISION?

And he gave him the covenant of circumcision: and so [Abraham] begat Isaac, and circumcised him the eighth day;

📖 Acts 7:8

Every penis has a foreskin. Circumcision involves removing the foreskin, which shields the head of the penis. In the United States, 60 percent of baby boys are circumcised, usually in the first few days or weeks after birth. Some parents choose circumcision because it's an important and ancient ritual, while others choose it because they believe it has health advantages.

Circumcision is a personal decision that you should make based on your own beliefs and after talking with your doctor. There is no clear medical evidence that circumcision provides health benefits for male babies. Circumcisions are painful and when parents are making the decision to expose their male children to circumcision, you should make an informed decision based on possible health benefits and risks, as well as cultural, religious, and ethnic traditions.

What are the pros and cons?

If there is no foreskin, it is easier to keep the head of the penis clean. however, you can just as easily pull the foreskin down over the head of the penis to keep it clean. It is true that bacteria can accumulate under the foreskin, which can lead to urinary tract infections. However the issue is cleanliness. Also, other arguments in favor of circumcision include concerns that an uncircumcised child will be seen as different from his friends or will feel different from his father who may be circumcised. Arguments against circumcision include the fact that the procedure is not medically necessary. Some parents believe circumcision is a form of mutilation that's painful and emotionally harmful to a child.

If we do decide to do it, what else should we know?

Expect the penis tip to be reddish or to secrete a yellowy liquid for a few days if you have your baby circumcised. Indications of infection: swelling or crusty, yellow sores containing cloudy liquid. If you suspect infection or if your baby has problems urinating—a trickling stream or expressions of discomfort—talk to your doctor immediately.

When should a circumcision be done?

Make it early, if at all. And talk the issue through with your doctor and spouse before the baby arrives—it's an emotionally charged issue and not to be confronted when you're fatigued from giving birth. Rather than having it done in the delivery room, wait a few hours or a few days. But delaying a circumcision until your baby is older than a few months can be traumatizing.

Keep in mind that there is no medical need for routine circumcision. There are baby boys who require a medical circumcision because the opening to the penis is either in the wrong place or the foreskin is too tight and will never stretch over the head of the penis. If this occurs, you physician will discuss your options with you.

60. DOES YOUR CHILD NEED A TONSILLECTOMY?

But mine eyes [are] unto thee, O GOD the Lord: in thee is my trust; leave not my soul destitute.

ꙮ Psalms 141:8

A tonsillectomy is a major surgical procedure and you should carefully consider your options before you subject your child to this procedure. Also, please note that just because your child gets their tonsils removed, it doesn't mean that your child will never get a sore throat again. A generation ago, tonsillectomies were performed almost routinely for enlarged tonsils and recurrent throat infections. However, only in the last few years have there been good long-term studies to show which children actually benefit from this surgery.

Currently, there are only a few reasons why a preschool-aged child might need a tonsillectomy:

- Surgery would be necessary and indeed urgent, if your child has very large tonsils that block the airway with symptoms of periodic stoppage of normal breathing during sleep.
- The tonsils would be removed right away if an abscess forms in one of the tonsils.
- A tonsillectomy may be recommended if your child has had more than seven episodes per year of strep throat or other substantial tonsil infections or if symptomatic tonsillitis did not resolve despite six months of antibiotic therapy.
- Children with loud snoring and restless sleeping may also benefit from removal of the tonsils and adenoids.

A tonsillectomy does not improve the health of children with allergies, ear infections, or recurrent minor upper respiratory infections. If both you and your physician feel that your child meets the criteria to benefit from a tonsillectomy, ask your primary care physician to refer you to an Ear, Nose and Throat doctor (ENT).

61. DEVELOPMENTAL MILESTONES— DON'T MISS THEM!

Train up a child in the way he should go; and when he is old, he will not depart from it.

༜ Proverbs 22:6

Your child's brain grows very fast both during the pregnancy and after birth. It is important to measure your child's development throughout their life, but more so in the first five years of life. Your child's development is measured by your doctor during the "Well Child" visits that are scheduled from birth to your child's fifth birthday. The schedule of visits are as follows:

First 10 days after birth	6 months of age	18 months of age
1 month of age	9 months of age	2 years
2 months of age	12 months of age	3 years
4 months of age	15 months of age	4–6 years

During these "Well Child" visits, your child's growth (height and weight) and development are assessed. When we talk about normal development, we are talking about developing skills in five important areas:

- **Gross motor:** using large muscle groups to sit, stand, walk, run, etc., keeping balance, and changing positions.
- **Fine motor:** using hands to be able to eat, draw, dress, play, write, and do many other things.
- **Language:** speaking, using body language and gestures, communicating, and understanding what others say.
- **Cognitive:** thinking skills, including learning, understanding, problem-solving, reasoning, and remembering.
- **Social:** interacting with others, having relationships with family, friends, and teachers, cooperating, and responding to the feelings of others.

During some of these "Well Child" visits, your child will also receive immunizations or baby shots. These "Well Child" visits are very important and you should take your child according to the schedule.

What are developmental milestones?

Developmental milestones are a set of functional skills or age-specific tasks that most children can do at a certain age range. Your pediatrician uses milestones to help check how your child's brain and muscles are developing. Although each milestone has an age level, the actual age when a normally developing child reaches each milestone can vary. Every child is unique!

62. WHY DO BABIES COME EARLY?

To everything there is a season, and a time to every purpose under the heaven; A time to be born, and a time to die; a time to plant, and a time to reap.

« Ecclesiastes 3: 1–2 »

A normal pregnancy lasts 40 weeks. When a baby is born before the 37th week, the baby is born prematurely. It takes 37–40 weeks for your baby's lungs, heart and brain to develop and be functional outside of the womb. Another important reason why your baby needs to be in the womb for 40 weeks is to gain the weight necessary to maintain their body heat and their ability to continue the development of their vital organs after birth. If a baby is born before the 37th week, babies have a difficult time eating enough to grow and maintaining their body temperatures. They also have immature lungs that don't function well outside of the womb.

Most mothers don't know in advance that their baby is going to be born prematurely, so when it happens, it comes as a great shock. There are several reasons why a woman might go into premature labor before her baby is sufficiently mature to cope with life outside the womb. These include:

- Infections. Urinary tract infections are the most common reason that a woman will go into premature labor. All women should drink eight glasses of water a day and when wiping, wipe front to back. That will help cut down the number of infections. If you are pregnant and think you might have a urinary tract infection, see your doctor immediately so that you can get treated properly.
- Smoking, stress or poor diet. (overeating, under-eating and eating the wrong foods). These three factors affect your blood vessels throughout your body and affect the blood vessels feeding the baby. If you smoke, the amount of oxygen available to the baby will be less. Also nicotine makes blood vessels constrict

and therefore decreases the amount of blood supply to the baby. Stress is thought to decrease the blood flow to the baby and also thought to increase the hormones in the mother that make the blood vessels spasm. Being overweight or being underweight is not good for either the mother or the baby. Diets high in fats and carbohydrates will clog the blood vessels feeding the baby.

- A multiple pregnancy, for example twins. The mother's womb can only grow so much and hold so much weight. If the womb is carrying more than one baby, there is a greater likelihood that the Mom will deliver early. However, most Moms can carry two babies to 37 weeks without a problem.

- Cervical incompetence. The cervix is the opening that the baby will come through. Some women have a cervix that doesn't stay closed in pregnancy, which will make the uterus contract as the baby grows. Your physician can stitch the cervix closed, which will help. One of the reasons you need to visit your OB/GYN provider is to check the competency or closure of the cervix.

- Life-threatening conditions such as pre-eclampsia. Pre-eclampsia is a medical condition that causes high blood pressure, kidney problems and liver problems. It can kill both the Mom and baby. The main indications that you may have pre-eclampsia are raised blood pressure and protein in your urine. This is the reason why your blood pressure and urine are checked at your OB/GYN appointments. Another sign is swelling in your feet, hands and face, especially if it comes up suddenly. However, some swelling is perfectly normal in pregnancy and on its own isn't necessarily a symptom of pre-eclampsia. In the early stages of the illness, women usually feel quite well. In the more advanced stages they may suffer severe headaches, flashing lights or spots before the eyes, sickness and pain in the upper part of the abdomen. It's possible that these symptoms may have other causes, which aren't dangerous, but as they could indicate serious pre-eclampsia, which needs urgent medical attention, you should contact your doctor immediately if you notice any of them

In some cases, you may never discover the reason why your baby was born prematurely. If you have had a previous premature birth, or if there is a possibility that you may have a premature baby again. The best way to guard against having your baby born too early, is to take care of yourself and to make sure you are getting prenatal care. You, the Mom, are the most important ingredient to make sure you have a healthy pregnancy and a healthy baby. Modern science can save a lot of babies born early. However, babies born early have a hard time catching up with their development. The best gift you can give your child is a healthy Mom, so take care of yourself.

63. MY KID HAS DIARRHEA—WHAT SHOULD I DO?

But Jesus said, Suffer little children, and forbid them not, to come unto me: for of such is the kingdom of heaven.

ᕓ Matthew 19:14

Normally, a child will have only one or two bowel movements per day, although a few more is normal if your child eats a lot of fruit and fiber. An occasional loose stool is nothing to worry about, but if your child's bowel movements *suddenly* change; that is, she or he poops more than normal and passes watery, mucus- or blood-streaked stools that are clear, yellow, green, or very dark, it's diarrhea.

Diarrhea, or frequent watery stools, is one of the more common childhood diseases. In the United States, most cases of diarrhea are relatively mild and are caused by a virus and don't pose a major health problem. When your child has diarrhea, the most important thing to do is to keep your child hydrated with liquids. When children get really sick from diarrhea it's primarily as a result of *dehydration*.

The most common causes of diarrhea are infections by a virus. When viruses infect your children they commonly do so through the intestines. The body then poops out the virus, which causes diarrhea. Other common causes of diarrhea are antibiotics or eating too much fruit or juice. Sometimes diarrhea can come from bacteria from food, which is food poisoning, an allergy to milk, or too much vitamin C. There are many names for diarrhea. One of the most common names is stomach flu. Stomach flu can be caused by either a virus or bacteria. When the stomach and/or intestine has the flu, they can't do their job, which will cause runny stools. Many different viruses can cause this condition. If your child has diarrhea accompanied by stomach cramps, vomiting, and a low fever, it's probably a form of gastroenteritis or stomach flu. *What's important here is to continue to give your child liquids so that your child will not become dehydrated. Diarrhea from the stomach flu is only dangerous if your child gets dehydrated. Give your child Pedialyte for 24 hours and lay off the milk for 24hours and then gradually add milk and bland foods depending on the age of your child.*

Some antibiotics can also cause diarrhea. . Antibiotics, especially the ones used to fight ear infections, can kill the "good" bacteria in your child's stomach, resulting in diarrhea. Talk to your pediatrician about alternatives, but basically, if your child needs to stay on the antibiotic, you would treat the diarrhea with Pedialyte for the first 24 hours and then gradually add milk and bland food depending on the age of your child.

Sugars or sugar substitutes can cause diarrhea. Too much juice or too many sweetened drinks in your child's diet may be causing your child's loose stools, so cutting back the amount of juice you give her should solve the problem in a week or so. Fruit juices containing sorbitol and high levels of fructose, such as pear juice, can upset a child's stomach.

Food poisoning can cause severe diarrhea with or without vomiting and accompanied by cramps, blood in the stool, and a fever. The most common causes for food poisoning is the bacteria E. coli. Other common causes for food poisoning are bacteria such as salmonella and shigella, but viruses can also cause food poisoning. If your child has these symptoms, you should have your pediatrician evaluate her and check a stool sample for bacterial infection. Sometimes these infections clear up on their own, but some, such as E. Coli infections, can be very serious if left untreated. Other than treating the bacteria with antibiotics, you treat the diarrhea with Pedialyte for the first day and then gradually add back milk and bland food depending on the age of the child.

You can buy Pedialyte in grocery stores and drug stores.

If your child is only on breast milk or formula, most pediatricians will add the milk back after the first 24 hours. In smaller children, such as babies, become dehydrated faster, so keep count of the number of poops your child has and call your doctor if your child has more than six poops or stops having wet diapers or no tears.

When your child has diarrhea, the American Academy of Pediatrics recommends that you call your pediatrician immediately if your child:

- Has diarrhea alternating with constipation
- Has blood in her stool
- Plays less than usual
- Urinates less than normal
- Parched, dry mouth
- Has sunken eyes
- Fewer tears when crying
- Has lost weight

You should also consult your pediatrician if your child refuses to eat or drink, has a fever that lasts longer than 24 hours, has blood in her stool, vomits up anything green or blood-tinged or that looks like coffee grounds, has severe abdominal pain, rash, jaundice or a swollen abdomen.

64. MY CHILD HAS FEVER—WHAT SHOULD I DO?

And he touched her hand, and the fever left her: and she arose, and ministered unto them.

                                                 ᏩᎦ Matthew 8:15

Fever is a rise in the body temperature significantly above the normal. A "normal body" temperature when taken with an oral thermometer is 98.6 ° F or 32° C. You can subtract a degree to this if you take the temperature rectally or add a degree to this if you take the temperature underneath the arm. So a normal temperature in a young child is about 99–100°F and parents should not be concerned unless the temperature climbs above that and stays there.

Fever is not a disease; instead, it is a symptom that can accompany many childhood illnesses, especially infections. Elevation in body temperature means different things at different ages. In general, you should call your pediatrician if your infant under three months of age has a rectal temperature above 100.4 F, if your infant aged 3–6 months has a temperature above 101 F, or if an infant above six months has a temperature above 103 F.

For most older children, it is not so much the number, but rather how your child is acting that is a concern. If your older child is alert, active and playful, is not having difficulty breathing, and is eating and sleeping well, or if the temperature comes down quickly with home treatments (and he is feeling well), then you don't necessarily need to call your doctor immediately.

However, it is important to keep in mind that a fever is not the only sign of a serious illness. While some older children are fine with a temperature of 104, others can be deathly ill with a temperature of 101 or even without a fever or a low temperature.

You should call your pediatrician or seek medical attention immediately if, in addition to fever, your child:

- is very irritable
- confused
- lethargic (doesn't easily wake up)
- has difficulty breathing
- has a rapid and weak pulse
- is refusing to eat or drink
- still appears ill, even after the fever is brought down,
- has a severe headache or other specific complaint (burning with urination, if he is limping, etc)
- or if he has a fever that persists for more than 24 to 48 hours.

Also, you should call your doctor if your child has a fever and another medical condition (heart disease, cancer, sickle cell, immune system problems, etc.).

When in doubt, call your doctor when your child has a fever, especially if you think that your child appears ill.

Treatment of a fever can include using an over-the-counter fever reducer, including products that contain acetaminophen (Tylenol) or ibuprofen (Motrin or Advil). If you child has an infection, *using a fever reducer will not help your child to get better any faster*, but they will probably make him feel better. The fever reducers only treat the fever. You should also give your child a lot of fluids when s/he has a fever, so that he does not get dehydrated. Keep in mind that treatment of a fever is usually to help your child feel better, so if he has a fever, but doesn't feel bad, especially if the fever is low grade, then you do not need to treat the fever. Do not give your children aspirin when they have a fever. Also when you give a fever reducer, wait 15 minutes before you take the temperature again. If the temperature is still elevated, sponge your child's chest and head with warm water and let the air dry the water off your child's body. This will gradually bring down the body's temperature. Never use cold water, as this will make your child shiver, which can drive up the core body temperature.

Is it safe to alternate acetaminophen and ibuprofen? If you are using the correct dosage of each medicine at the correct times, then it is probably safe in most children, although there is no research to prove that it helps or that it is safe. The problem is that it is easy to get confused and give an extra dose of one or the other medicines. And in some children, especially if they are dehydrated or have other medical problems, giving both medications can cause serious side effects, especially with the kidneys. If you are alternating fever reducers, then write down a schedule with the times that you are giving the medicines so that the correct medicine is always given at the correct time.

Things to remember when your child has a fever:

- Never ignore any fever in an infant under three.
- Never give your child a sponge bath with cold water and never give your child a sponge bath with alcohol.

65. HEY MOM, DID YOUR BABY GET HER SHOTS?

He will not allow your foot to slip; He who keeps you will not slumber.

ൟ Psalm 121:3

Regular checkups at your pediatrician's office or local health clinic are an important way to keep children healthy. During these visits, one of the services that your baby should get is immunizations or Baby Shots, which will provide the best available defense against many dangerous childhood diseases. Immunizations or Baby Shots protect children against: hepatitis B, polio, measles, mumps, rubella (German measles), pertussis (whooping cough), diphtheria, tetanus (lockjaw), *Haemophilus influenzae* type b, pneumococcal infections, and chickenpox. All of these immunizations need to be given before your baby is two years old in order for them to be protected.

Some parents take their babies to the Health Department for their Baby Shots and to the Pediatrician for other services. If your baby gets their Baby Shots at the local health department, make sure that you take the Baby Shot record to the doctor's office every time you go. Giving your baby too many Baby Shots is just as harmful as not getting the Baby shots at all.

Keep track of your child's immunizations—it's the only way you can be sure your child is up-to-date. Also, check with your pediatrician or health clinic at each visit to find out if your child needs any booster shots or if any new vaccines have been recommended since this schedule was prepared.

Remember! Always give your baby's doctor the record of Baby Shots that your child has been given

SECTION VI

THE ROLE OF MENTAL HEALTH ON LONGEVITY

66. EXERCISE FOR BETTER HEALTH

Seest thou how faith wrought with his works, and by works was faith made perfect?"

ᐧ James 2:22

You do not have to be a trained athlete to enjoy the benefits of exercise. A walk around the mall every day can help burn off excess fat and keep the heart, lungs, muscles and bones in good shape.

Regular exercise improves the way you look and feel, and gives you more of the endurance and energy you need to live an active life. Best of all, it slows down the aging process. Exercise helps keep the body in tune. It improves the circulation in the heart and muscles, and helps maintain the thickness of bones so they will not break so easily.

Exercise can do you more good than any fad diet. A two hundred-pound woman who wants to lose one pound can do so without cutting down on food if she walks for three miles. At that rate, with a little perseverance and regularity, she can walk herself to a healthier weight.

As if such benefits weren't enough, exercise also helps relieve stress. Ask anyone who does it. You'll be talking to a believer.

When you exercise, drink enough water, especially on hot days. You lose fluids when you exercise, and if you don't replace them, it is possible to get heat exhaustion and heat stroke. *If you are doing vigorous exercise and you feel faint, lightheaded, dizzy, have a headache or feel thirsty, stop at once and drink some water.*

Every so often, we hear about someone who died because he or she had heart disease and over-exerted. You can avoid this by getting a physical exam, and following your doctor's advice about how much and what kind of exercise is right for you. There is no evidence that physically active people are more likely to have heart attacks than inactive people are. Just take it easy, and don't overdo it. Little by little you'll get stronger and have more stamina.

If you *do* feel discomfort in your chest during exercise, stop and contact your doctor. Especially if you have not exercised in a long time, start slowly and gradually increase how much you do. That way you'll avoid injury to your joints and muscles.

67. COMMON MYTHS ABOUT EXERCISE

Ye see then how that by works a man is justified, and not by faith only.
∾ James 2:24

People resist exercise because they think it will be too hard or because they are overweight. But the fact is, almost anyone can exercise. Thirty minutes a day, is all you need. And one of the best exercises you can do is walking. It is easy, requires no equipment except a good pair of walking shoes, and which most people find very pleasant once they get into it. Each day that you walk, your body becomes a little bit healthier. Before long, you'll also notice that you are becoming stronger and have more endurance.

Here are some common myths about exercise, and some proven truths:

- Myth #1: Exercise makes you feel tired. The truth is that as you get in shape, exercising makes you more energetic. Regular exercise can also help you to resist fatigue and handle stress better.
- Myth #2: Exercise takes too long. The truth is that tremendous benefits from regular exercise can be achieved with only 30 minutes of exercise every day.
- Myth #3: All exercise gives you the same benefits. The truth is that, while all physical exercise gives enjoyment, regular and sustained exercise, like walking, jogging, bicycling and swimming have benefits for your heart and lungs. Weight lifting does not have the same benefits as swimming. Actually, lifting heavy weights raises blood pressure. In general, basketball players and swimmers live longer than football players and weight lifters.
- Myth #4: The older you are, the less exercise you need. The truth is that we all tend to become less active as we get older. Since everyone can benefit from regular exercise, it is impor-

tant to sustain a high level of activity even when we are tempted to sit back and rest on our laurels. The important thing is to tailor your exercise program to your ability and fitness level.

- Myth #5: You have to be athletic to exercise. The truth is that most exercise does not require any particular skill or training. You simply need to move your muscles vigorously for 30 minutes every day. Many people who find organized sports difficult do very well when they find something like walking that they can excel in.

Commit to something, even if it's simply taking a walk with a friend for thirty minutes each day.

Just do it!

68. HOW TO REDUCE THE STRESS IN YOUR LIFE

Whom we preach, warning every man, and teaching every man in all wisdom; that we may present every man perfect in Christ Jesus.

◈ Colossians 1:28

Stress is a fact of life we can't change. But your attitude about stress can change catastrophe into opportunity. Yes, stress can be made into a positive experience. Positive stress can provide creativity to solve problems, energy to perform tasks, or staying power to get the job done. It can bring out the best in us.

Your attitude about stress can change catastrophe into opportunity.

Destructive stress is stress we experience because we feel we have no control over a situation. Destructive stress helps bring on heart disease, cancer, ulcers, and many other diseases.

Here is how you can reduce the destructive stress in your life

- *Have a Positive Attitude!* Alcoholics Anonymous has a saying: "Try and think of what was worrying you two weeks ago." Most of us can't remember because the problem or irritation got fixed. Sometimes our impatience is what causes the trouble. We may feel we're in the middle of a crisis just because we don't know how to get out of a stressful experience today. So practice patience.
- *Have a Plan B.* Know in advance what you will do if your present plan doesn't work. Having a parachute gives you the confidence to take risks.
- *Don't over-commit yourself.* You can't do it all, be everywhere, or be all things to all people.

- *Know your limits.* A day only has twenty-four hours. You can't pack thirty hours into twenty-four hours, no matter how hard you try.
- *Develop the courage to be imperfect and still feel good about yourself.* We all look foolish, sound dumb, and make stupid decisions at times. Making mistakes is a part of living. Only God is perfect.
- *Accept the fact that people will disappoint you, especially your children and others who are special to you.* They are not in this world to live up to your expectations.
- *Don't expect everyone to be fair and reasonable.* Every cloud has a silver lining. Be creative and find it. Even in the best of circumstances there is a down side. But don't curse because roses have thorns. Instead, celebrate because thorn bushes have roses.
- *Just say "No" and mean it.* From time to time, people will make unreasonable demands on you, ask you to do things you do not want to do. You are not in this world to live up to everyone's demands.
- *Accept the fact that things won't always work out the way you want.* Baseball stars make millions of dollars per year and they are lucky to get a hit two out of ten times at bat. Learn to forgive yourself, appreciate and love yourself. After all, that is the greatest love of all.

69. HOW TO RELAX

A cheerful heart is a good medicine, but a downcast spirit dries up the bones.

അ Proverbs 17:22

Do you need to settle your nerves? That doesn't have to mean Caribbean islands or expansive spas. Relaxation is a state of mind and of lifestyle. Everyone can relax by just following a few simple rules. That doesn't mean that you'll never feel stressed—only that you'll know how to handle stress, and have fewer occasions to be irritated and short tempered. Here are the rules:

- Don't purposely put yourself in stressful situations. When possible, avoid situations and people that upset you.
- Tell yourself a joke. Blow a stressful situation out of proportion to emphasize the absurdity. If you are stuck in traffic, just imagine what it would be like to be stuck there for ten years. By then, your children will be adults and married. If you are lucky, you will miss their teenage years altogether.
- Sigh a lot and take deep breaths. When you breathe in, push in on your stomach and hold it in. When you can no longer hold it, let go very slowly.
- Listen to music you enjoy.
- Imagine looking at a waterfall and watch your worries wash away. Or imagine yourself as a millionaire, the President, or a knight in shining armor.
- Walk away from a stressful situation. Take a fifteen-minute walk and swing your arms. As you do, pretend a helium balloon is holding up your head.
- Talk with friends, but only confide in someone who has your best interests at heart. If you do not have someone to talk to, write a letter to someone or just write out your problems. Talk into a tape recorder if you have one.

- Make an "appointment" to deal with the problem at another time. Often, you'll find that in an hour or a day, the problem just isn't a problem anymore
- Take a hot bath—learn from the Japanese, they live longer than anyone else in the world. If you want a quick fix for stress, follow up the hot bath with a very cold shower.
- Learn to use exercise as stress relief. In any case, move your muscles. Play a game, run, skip, and just get out of the house. If you feel violent, take it out on your mattress. Hit it as hard as you want, it will not complain. Avoid watching TV, and by all means get out of bed.

Alcohol and drugs only make things worse!!!

70. LAUGHTER IS GOOD MEDICINE

For our heart shall rejoice in him, because we have trusted in his holy name."

☙ Psalm 33: 21

The song says: *When you laugh, the world laughs with you,
                   when you cry, you cry all alone.*

Actually, there is nothing wrong with either laughing or crying. They are expressions of honest human emotions that can make you feel less frustrated and less angry. Crying is a way of letting the hurt out. Even people of great faith, like King David, knew the power of lamentation. A laugh, on the other hand, is like sunshine on a cloudy day. Life without laughter is dreary. An honest laugh cheers us. It is the music, the gospel chorus of our conversations. Laughter among friends is the glue that holds people together. Victor Hugo said, "I like laughter that opens the lips and the heart, and reveals at the same time, the pearls of the soul."

In his book, *Laughter is the Best Medicine,* Dr. Norman Vincent Peale explains that certain disease ailments respond to a healthy emotional attitude, which can be prompted by laughter. The writer Norman Cousins has similarly described how he helped himself recover from cancer by watching old Chaplin movies and videos of Sid Caesar shows.

Scientists are now discovering that laughter and a positive attitude can increase the release of endorphins and promote the manufacture of T-cells. Endorphins make us feel good and decrease our sensitivity to pain. T-cells act like sentinels in our blood to remove harmful microorganisms and cells. (Chronic depression can actually weaken your immune system and lower your endorphin level.)

When you laugh, electrical impulses are triggered and chemicals released into your blood stream that dull pain and tranquilize the soul. Other substances that are released with laughter improve digestion, make the blood vessels relax to improve circulation, and lower blood pressure.

A philosopher said over a hundred years ago, "Laughter is the most healthful exercise. It is one of the greatest helps to digestion with which I am acquainted. It stirs up the blood, expands the chest, electrifies the nerves and clears away the cobwebs from the brain. It is the cheapest luxury man enjoys."

71. HOW MUCH SLEEP IS ENOUGH?

We are the new man, which is renewed in knowledge after the image of Him that created us.

ᕉ Colossians 3:10 "

Obviously, we need our sleep. In fact, if you live to be ninety years old, you probably will have spent thirty years of it asleep. Sleep refreshes us and restores our vigor. But no one is sure how that works. The obvious answer would be that our bodies and brains need the rest, but in fact, our brain, organs, and muscles are very much awake twenty-four hours a day.

As you first fall asleep, your brain, along with your blood pressure, heart rate, and body temperature, all slow down and you fall into what is know as *slow wave sleep*. About an hour-and-a-half later, you enter a dream phase, called REM sleep. REM stands for rapid eye movement. Not only do your eyes move rapidly in this phase, but your blood pressure, pulse, and respiration also act erratically. In this state, your brain is as active as when you are awake.

Some people do very well with three hours of sleep and others need ten hours to feel refreshed. It's said that Einstein slept twelve hours a night. Infants sleep up to eighteen hours per day. As we get older, we require less sleep.

Some people can't sleep when they want to. The most common reasons for insomnia are:

- Traveling to a different time zone
- Annoying noises
- Uncomfortable mattresses
- Physical ailments
- Pain
- Drug side effects
- Irregular working hours
- Napping during the day
- Worries, anxiety, and depression.

Some people have trouble falling asleep because of emotional problems that can be corrected with counseling. Still others only imagine that they do not get enough sleep. Under observation, insomniacs often get more sleep than they think they do.

Sleeping pills often make insomnia worse in the end. Most sleeping pills make you miss the most restful sleep cycles and take away your dreams. Don't let anything or anyone take away your dreams! The best ways to improve your sleeping habits are to:

- Avoid naps.
- Exercise during the day so you will be tired at night.
- Avoid watching hyperactive TV shows before you go to sleep.
- Count cows, sheep, or the hairs on the back of your neck.
- Learn to meditate

If you still have trouble, talk to your doctor. He or she may help you discover what's keeping you awake, and may also be able to suggest remedies.

72. THE HEALING POWER OF LOVE

Beloved, let us love one another, for love is of God; and everyone who loves is born of God and knows God. He who does not love does not know God, for God is love.

∞ 1 John 4: 7, 9

Love and intimacy affect not only the quality of our lives but our very survival. Lonely, depressed and isolated people are much more likely to develop serious illnesses or to die prematurely than those who keep close ties with friends, relatives, and club, church and community members. Dean Ornish, M.D., founder of Preventive Medicine Research Institute, states that he is not aware of any aspect of our health–not diet, not smoking, not exercise, not stress, not genetics, not drugs, not surgery–that does more to protect us from the likelihood of illness and premature death than the healing power of love and intimacy.

By love, we mean anything that makes us feel intimately connected with others, part of a community, small or large. That love can be romantic, but it can also be spiritual or religious. It works in all things, great and small. We get warmth from the ties that hold us to other human beings. We get warmth even from the love that goes on between a pet, and us or, sometimes, by just looking up at the sky.

People these days are so caught up in their jobs, their computers, their videos and electronic games that they don't find the time to spend with friends or even family. But spending quality time with friends and family is a necessity, not a luxury. Our need for love and intimacy is as important as eating, sleeping and breathing.

Love comes to those who give it. You can know love by hugging a friend or a child (especially a baby), kissing a mother, embracing a friend. Maybe love means rubbing your father's feet, telling your grandparents that you love them, or writing your brother a letter telling him how much you appreciate him—these are all ways of sharing love. We can spread love by small acts of kindness, such as opening a door for a stranger.

If you aren't experiencing the love you need, know that to love others and be loved you must first love yourself. Start at home and tell yourself how much you love yourself and let your love grow. The world is waiting!

73. BEAT DRUMS AND NOT EACH OTHER

Now Cain talked with Abel his brother and it came to pass.
When they were in the field, that Cain rose up against Abel
His brother and killed him.

ॐ Genesis 4:8

On average, sixty-five people each day die from interpersonal violence, and more than 6,000 are physically injured. An estimated 1,000 to 2,000 children die each year from physical abuse. Violence has a high cost to you, your family and our community. The average costs of medical and mental health treatment, emergency medical response, productivity losses, health insurance, and disability payments for the victims of injuries are estimated at $34 billion, with lost quality of life estimated at an additional $145 billion. People who act violently are usually victims of violence themselves.

There are lots of theories as to why we are violent with one another. Some people become violent because they want what you have and feel that they should be able to take it. Some people become violent as a means of making others do what they want. Sometimes loved ones are violent with each other out of misplaced passion. One group of people may be violent toward another group in order to exert control. At the base of all violence, however, is frustration.

Whatever the reason, at the root of all violence is selfishness, "I want what I want when I want it." That feeling of false entitlement occurs in violent acts toward women at the hands of men, it occurs when one racial group feels it needs to control another racial group, and it occurs when a thief takes what doesn't belong to him or her.

It will take all of us working together to address the epidemic of violence that exits in our country. One of the practical things we can do is to limit the amount of violence that enters our homes and the minds of our young people through the television, movies and video games. Another thing we can do is to give each other the benefit of the doubt and also forgive each other. A wise man once said, "If a man hits you on one cheek then turn and offer the next cheek." This is easier said than done. However, each of us can do a little each day to reduce the amount of violence in our lives.

As John Lennon said, "Let's give peace a chance!"

74. I THINK I'M DEPRESSED—WHAT SHOULD I DO?

Peace I leave with you, my peace I give unto you: not as the world giveth, give I unto you. Let not your heart be troubled, neither let it be afraid.

☙ John 14:27

All of us at times feel like the world is closing in on us. We all get blue, sad and down in the dumps because of things that happen to us. We usually say we are "depressed" when situational problems affect us and we don't have a clear solution to our problems. Although we state that we are "depressed"; most of us find the inner strength to keep on moving and eventually find solutions to our problems and develop a brighter outlook. Although you feel sad at the time of the situation if you are able to remain focused on your daily living and work, your "depression" is normal and situational and probably does not need intervention by a health care professional.

There is a different type of depression that affects about one in twenty Americans. Over 11 million people get depressed every year. Depression affects twice as many women as men and is becoming a growing problem in the teenage. Depression is not just "feeling blue" or "down in the dumps." It is more than being sad or feeling grief after a loss. This depression, we'll call it medical depression, is a medical disorder (just like diabetes, high blood pressure, or heart disease are medical disorders) that day after day affects your thoughts, feelings, physical health, and behaviors.

Medical depression may be caused by many things, including:

- Family history and genetics.
- Other general medical illnesses.
- Certain medicines.
- Drugs or alcohol.
- Other psychiatric conditions.

Certain life conditions (such as extreme stress, or grief) may bring on a depression or prevent a full recovery. In some people, depression occurs even when life is going well. Depression is not your fault. It is not a weakness. It is a medical illness. Depression is treatable.

How will I know if I am depressed?

People who have major depressive disorder have a number of symptoms nearly every day, all day, for at least two weeks. These always include at least one of the following:

- Loss of interest in things you used to enjoy.
- Feeling sad, blue, or down in the dumps.
- Feeling slowed down or restless and unable to sit still.
- Feeling worthless or guilty.
- Increase or decrease in appetite or weight.
- Thoughts of death or suicide.
- Problems concentrating, thinking, remembering, or making decisions.
- Trouble sleeping or sleeping too much.
- Loss of energy or feeling tired all of the time.
- With depression, there are often other physical or psychological symptoms, including:
- Headaches.
- Other aches and pains.
- Digestive problems.
- Sexual problems.
- Feeling pessimistic or hopeless.
- Being anxious or worried.

What should I do if I feel depressed?

Too often people do not get help for their depression because they don't recognize the symptoms, have trouble asking for help, blame themselves, or don't know that treatments are available.

Family practitioners, clinics, or health maintenance organizations are often the first places that people go for help. These health care providers will:

- Find out if there is a physical cause for your depression.
- Treat the depression.
- Refer you to a mental health specialist for further evaluation and treatment.

If you do not have a regular health care provider, contact your local health department, community mental health clinic, or hospital. University medical centers also provide treatment for depression.

How will treatment help me?

Treatment reduces the pain and suffering of depression. Successful treatment removes the symptoms of depression and returns you to your normal life. The earlier you get treated for your depression, the sooner you will begin to feel better. As with other medical illnesses, the longer you have the depression before you seek treatment, the more difficult it can be to treat.

Most people who are treated for depression feel better and return to daily activities in several weeks. Because it takes several weeks for treatment to work, it is important to get treatment early before your depression gets worse.

As with any medical condition, you may have to try one or two treatments before finding the best one. It is important not to get discouraged if the first treatment does not work. In almost every case, there is a treatment for the depression that will work for you.

What type of treatment will I get?

The major treatments for depression are:

- Antidepressant medicine.
- Psychotherapy.
- Antidepressant medicine combined with psychotherapy.
- The love and affection of your family and friends.

SECTION VII

LIFESTYLES THAT
SHORTEN YOUR LIFE

75. CIGARETTE SMOKING AND
YOUR HEALTH

Neither give place to the devil. . . .

怕 Ephesians 4:27

Cigarette smoking is addictive and dangerous to your health. Tobacco use is responsible for nearly one in five deaths in the United States—420,000 deaths annually. Smoking and chewing tobacco are major causes of heart disease and many cancers. Smoking may also cause chronic bronchitis and emphysema. During pregnancy, smoking may cause damage to the unborn baby. Children living with smokers have more respiratory disorders, such as bronchitis and asthma.

Passive smoking, which means inhaling someone else's smoke, causes 5,000 deaths a year from lung cancer and heart disease. Smoking also:

- Makes your clothes and hair smell
- Wrinkles your skin
- Wastes your money
- Makes a chimney out of your nose
- Tells the world that you do not have control over your behavior
- Make non-smokers stay away from you
- Stains your teeth
- Makes food tasteless
- Makes you cough
- Makes your breath stink (You miss a lot of hugs and kisses when you smoke.)

If you smoke and want to stop, you should know that people who stop cold turkey are more successful than people who try to stop gradually. It's true that the more you smoked the harder it is to stop, but you *can* stop. You just have to decide to. If you need a little help, your doctor can prescribe nicotine delivered via patches, gum or nasal spray. Some people find it easier to kick the habit by slowly decreasing their dose in this way.

Just one year after you stop smoking, your risk of a heart attack declines sharply, to the same level as a non-smoker's.

You owe it to yourself and your family to give up this addictive drug. We need to train our children not to smoke just as we educate and counsel them on the dangers of other hard drugs.

Remember: The Surgeon General of the United States warns that cigarette smoking is harmful to you and can cause death.

Don't let your life go up in smoke!

76. ALCOHOL MAKES YOU A BAD LIVER

Wine is a mocker, strong drink a brawler; and whoever is led astray by it is not wise.

ᐤ Proverbs 20:1

A little alcohol per day is not harmful. In the story of the miracle of Canaan, Jesus turned water into wine so the wedding guests could enjoy themselves. He even suggested that wine could settle the stomach.

But problems arise when we drink too much. Alcohol can make us lose control and become abusive. Alcohol is also an addictive chemical that can be harmful to our health.

In the United States, alcohol consumption has gone down in the general population, but not among African-American men, among whom there has been an increase in alcohol-related death and disability. People who drink heavily rely on alcohol for nourishment and lose their appetite for wholesome food, so they also suffer from malnutrition.

A six-pack of beer or three shots of whiskey a day for ten years will cause cirrhosis of the liver. *Cirrhosis* describes what happens to the liver when alcohol or other chemicals cause the normal tissue to be replaced with scar tissue, so that the liver can no longer do its job as the cleansing agent of the blood.

Cirrhosis of the liver is not reversible. But with good treatment it can be stabilized– *if* the patient stops drinking alcohol and follows a good diet. If you have these symptoms, the simple message is to stop drinking and seek medical treatment. If you drink heavily and do not have these symptoms, STOP while you are still healthy. Why take a chance on this deadly disease?

While we can survive without alcohol, we can't survive without our liver. With a healthy liver, you can be a long liver, but you can't be a long liver with a bad liver.

77. ALCOHOL AND YOUR BRAIN

For the drunkard and the glutton will come to poverty, and drowsiness will clothe a man with rags.

೨ Proverb 23:21

Alcohol is a major contributor to accidents, drowning, violence, and sexual assaults. There is also good evidence that people who drink too much alcohol are likely to abuse street drugs as well.

Every drink of alcohol destroys brain cells. For moderate drinkers, that loss isn't serious. We have several billion brain cells and we can do very nicely with a few million less. But for an alcoholic, the loss can be critical.

Have you ever had a long talk with someone, but when you say hello the next morning, he or she doesn't remember talking to you? Short-term memory is the first thing to go with alcoholics. Once brain cells are lost, they can never be replaced. Loss of brain cells also contribute to senility.

Protect your brain and your brainpower–don't drink too much.

78. DRINKING AND DRIVING DON'T MIX

Let us walk properly, as in the day, not in revelry and drunkenness, not in licentiousness and lewdness, not in strife and envy.

ᕷ Romans 13:13

When we think about drinking and driving, the driver is certainly at risk. But there can be more than one victim when a person who has been drinking drives. Drinking alcohol produces poor judgment and slower reaction time. People under the influence of alcohol can feel elated and over-confident. They may drive faster and take risks that they would not ordinarily take. If they take such risks while you're walking or driving near them, you can become a victim.

You can also become a victim by sitting in the passenger's seat of a of a drunk person's car. This advice holds especially true for teenagers and young adults who like to go to bars. When Willie Sutton, the bank robber, was asked why he robbed banks, he replied: "That's where the money is." Well, bars are where the alcohol is, and even if the young person is not drinking, he or she will be around many people who are. Warn your children not only that they should not drink and drive, but they should also not be in a car with someone who has been drinking. They are at risk of being involved in accident.

Warn your children not only that they should not drink and drive, but they should also not be in a car with someone who has been drinking.

Be a friend to your kids, spouse, neighbor and yourself. Speak out against mixing drinking with driving.

79. BUCKLE UP FOR SAFETY

My people are destroyed for lack of knowledge.

ᔥ Hosea 4:6

It should trouble us all to see children riding in cars driven by adults, and neither the adult nor the child has a seat belt on. The popular press and television have stressed the importance of seat belts and air bags for the past ten years, yet some Americans foolishly ignore the laws as well their children's and their own safety.

A car is a 2000–pound weapon. Even at thirty miles per hour, if you have to stop suddenly, anything in the car that is loose becomes a flying object or missile. You yourself may have had the experience of stopping suddenly, so that the purse or grocery bag next to you on the passenger seat hit the floor. Now think of your child sitting or even standing in that seat. If the child isn't protected by a seat belt, he or she will fall to the floor just as the groceries did, or, worse, fly into the windshield.

You need the same protection as your child. If you have to stop suddenly and do not have your seat belt on, your chest will slam into the steering wheel and your head into the windshield. Car accidents may not be avoidable but such injuries can be avoided.

Here are some common reasons people do not wear seat belts, and the facts these people fail to see:

- *I am not going far.* Most accidents occur within two miles from home.
- *My clothes will wrinkle.* Take off your suit coat while you are driving. In any case, it is better to have wrinkled clothes than to be injured.
- *The shoulder harness chokes me.* Most cars allow you to adjust the shoulder harness.
- *It is okay that my children do not wear seat belts if they are in the back seat.* Princess Diana was in the back seat of her car

when it crashed. She died of massive internal bleeding from the impact against the back seat.

- *Wearing seat belts is a hassle.* Recovering from injuries, not to mention funeral expenses, is far more of a hassle.

When you come right down to it, there is no good reason not to wear your seat belt while driving.

---

80. SEX AND RESPONSIBILITY

Do not fret because of evil men or be envious of those who do wrong. For like the grass, they will soon wither. . . . Trust the Lord and do good.

ॐ Psalm 37:1–3

More and more people are getting sexually transmitted diseases, and they are getting them at younger and younger ages. Thirteen- and fourteen-year-olds, without even the basic understanding of safe sex, are engaging in sexual activities and are being infected by diseases.

Sex is not an activity that should be taken lightly. In fact, sex can and does kill. It kills not only with HIV/AIDS but in other ways as well. If you're too young to have a baby, your chance of severe complications is high.

When young people have babies as a byproduct of unprotected sex, they have just committed themselves to responsibilities likely to hurt their education, their ability to make a living for themselves and their offspring, and even their ability to mature into adulthood appropriately. This is why it is so important that we teach ourselves and our children to act responsibly when we make decisions regarding sexual intercourse.

If we, as parents, carry out our sexual lives in an irresponsible manner, it should be no surprise when our children mimic our behavior. The culture, too, plays a strong role. If our children are bombarded at an early age with sexually explicit videos and TV, they are more likely to experiment at a younger age with sex. Children who experiment with sex at young ages are also more prone to develop sexually transmitted diseases or become pregnant due to unsafe sexual practices.

We all have the responsibility to approach sex with respect and caution. The marriage environment is an optimal sexual environment, where two people committed to having sex with only each other, are also responsible enough to bring babies into their lives. Sex outside of a monogamous relationship can be fraught with serious consequences. If you decide to have sex outside of a committed relationship, do the responsible thing and wear a condom, whether you are a man or woman. Condoms effectively prevent the spread of sexually transmitted diseases such as gonorrhea, syphilis and HIV. DO the right thing and be responsible.

81. WHAT IS HIV?

For ye were sometimes darkness, but now are ye light in the Lord; walk as children of the Light!

         ∽ Ephesians 5:8

HIV, Human Immunodeficiency Virus, is a virus that attacks our body's ability to fight infections and cancer. Everyone infected with HIV can develop AIDS, but the length of time between being infected with HIV and developing AIDS varies by person and the health of the person. Those people who stay healthy and take the AIDS medication, often live very long disease-free lives.

This virus has gotten more widespread since the early 1970s, and today it infects about 1 million Americans. African Americans only make up 13 percent of the US population but account for 40 percent of Americans that are infected and affected with HIV/AIDS. HIV/AIDS is among the top three causes of death for African-American men aged 25–54 years and among the top four causes of death for African-American women aged 20–54 years old. It was the number one cause of death for African-American women aged 25–34 years old.

The good news about this virus is that you can actually prevent yourself from getting it. It's not like the flu virus or a common cold virus, which infects large groups of people each year through airborne transmission. The virus known as HIV can only infect you if you let it, through unsafe sexual practices or from infected needles.

You can also get HIV from blood or blood products of persons infected with the HIV virus. Blood banks are now very good at ensuring that all donated blood is free of the HIV virus, so today the virus is rarely if ever transmitted through blood transfusion. People who get blood-borne HIV usually get it by sharing dirty needles and syringes contaminated by the HIV virus. When IV drug users who have HIV share their needles with other people, those other people are likely to get the HIV virus.

The HIV virus is transmitted through body fluids. Latex condoms are a good barrier against the transmission of HIV during the sex act.

Mothers who are infected with the HIV virus will expose their unborn children to the virus. Some of these babies go on to develop the HIV infection and AIDS as well, but some babies born to mothers who are HIV positive do not develop AIDS.

You are not likely to become infected with HIV if you avoid unprotected sexual intercourse and don't share dirty needles.

82. WHAT IS AIDS?

Trust in the Lord and He will make your righteousness shine like the dawn, and justice of your cause like the noonday sun.

AIDS stands for Acquired Immune Deficiency Syndrome. Often, an HIV infected person receives a diagnosis of AIDS after developing one of the diseases associated with the HIV virus. An HIV positive person can also be diagnosed as having AIDS without having one of the AIDS related disease, if the number of T-cells is low. T-cells help fight disease and when those cells are low, our bodies can't fight off bacteria, viruses or cancer cells.

A positive HIV test result does not mean that a person has AIDS. A diagnosis of AIDS is made by a physician using certain clinical criteria, such as the T-cell count and the presence of one of the diseases associated with AIDS.

Infection with HIV can weaken the immune system to the point that it has difficulty fighting off certain infections. These types of infections are known as "opportunistic" infections, because they take advantage of a weakened immune system to cause illness.

Many of the infections that cause problems for people with AIDS and may be life-threatening are determined by the health of the individual and the individual's immune system. The immune system, of a person with AIDS is weakened to the point that medical intervention may be necessary to prevent or treat a serious illness.

Today there are medical treatments that can slow down the rate at which HIV weakens the immune system. There are other treatments that can prevent or cure some of the illnesses associated with AIDS. As with other diseases, early detection offers more options for treatment and preventive care.

If you are infected with the HIV virus, it is important to take your medications so that you can slow down the progression of the infection. A stronger immune system will help you enjoy a higher quality of life.

83. INFECTIOUS HEPATITIS

Bless the Lord, O my soul, And forget not all His benefits: Who forgives all your iniquities, Who heals all your diseases, Who redeems your life from destruction, Who crowns you with loving kindness and tender mercies, Who satisfies your mouth with good things, So that your youth is renewed like the eagle's.

ᛞ Psalm 103:2–5

Hepatitis A is caused by a virus that damages the cells of the liver. It spreads by close contact either with an infected person or by drinking or eating foods that contain the virus. It takes two to six weeks after the exposure for the infected person to get sick.

When hepatitis A strikes, the patient will feel tired, have stomach pain, lose their appetite, feel like vomiting, and generally feel lousy. The urine may also be as dark as Coca-Cola, and fever will occur that generally disappears within the first few days. The most common sign is jaundice, which is a yellowing of the skin and of the whites of the eyes.

If you have these symptoms, contact your doctor immediately. Only a physician will know for sure if you have hepatitis. In the meantime, avoid close contact with others so that you will not spread the disease.

Children usually develop only mild cases of the disease and get better within one to two weeks. Hepatitis A strikes harder in adults and recovery takes up to six weeks.

If you contract hepatitis, a physician can shorten your recovery period and, possibly, prevent a relapse. The treatment most often is bed rest and proper diet. In time, you will be as good as new. To prevent the infection in the first place, wash your hands often, avoid close contact with strangers, and be careful about what you put in your mouth.

A public health approach to hepatitis is vaccination for those at risk and gamma globulin injections for those who have been exposed to hepatitis A.

SECTION VIII

LIVING WITH
THE BIG "C"

84. CANCER: MYTHS AND FACTS

Your body is the temple–the very sanctuary–of the Holy Ghost, who lives with you, Whom you have received (as a Gift) from God.

သာ 1 Corinthians 6:19

Cancer is the second leading cause of death in the United States, yet only 50 percent of African-American women get Pap tests, and only one-out-of-five get regular mammograms, rectal, or breast exams. For the past thirty years, the rate of death from cancer has been decreasing for White American but increasing for African Americans.

Some cancers can be related to your genes, but several types of cancers can be avoided. What we eat and drink, as well as where we live and work, can decide our fate.

Freedom begins with knowing the facts. Too many of us "know" things about cancer that simply aren't true:

Myth # 1: Cancer is an illness that mostly White people get.
Fact: Cancer death occurs ten years earlier in African Americans than in Whites. An important reason for this is that African-American patients often are not diagnosed early enough.

Early diagnosis and timely treatment can make all the difference.

Myth # 2: Cancer is fatal. Once somebody gets it, it is over.
Fact: One-out-of-two White Americans who have cancer are completely cured, but only one out of three African-American patients are as fortunate. Don't ignore or deny obvious signs and symptoms of cancer. The key to cancer's cure is early detection and treatment. Do not wait for pain, because that may be too late.

Here are the signs you must know. See a doctor at once if you have:

- Been spitting up blood
- Blood in your stool or if your stool is black in color
- A mole or wart that changed colors or got bigger
- Been feeling tired and have lost weight without trying
- Persistent headaches, blurred vision or weakness in one of your limbs
- A sore that does not heal
- Difficulty swallowing, hoarseness, or cough not related to a cold
- An unexplained lump in any part of your body

Cancer is a reality for many Americans. Don't get caught up with myths of home remedies. The facts about cancer prevention could save your life. By seeing your doctor for an annual check-up or if you or a loved one has any of the danger signs we've listed, you can help doctors and researchers in their fight against cancer. You may also be saving a precious life.

85. PREVENTING CANCER

It is neither good to eat meat or drink wine nor do anything by which your brother stumbles or is offended or made weak.

ᏧᏩ Romans 14:21

What you put in your mouth has a lot to do with your risk of developing cancer. The American Cancer Society has targeted good nutrition, along with the avoidance of tobacco, as the best ways to prevent cancer. A low fat diet may reduce your risk of breast cancer, and not smoking certainly reduces your risk for lung cancer and other forms of cancer, along with heart disease. Supplementing your diet with vitamins A and E may also reduce your chances of getting lung cancer, and eating foods high in fiber and calcium may prevent colon cancer.

Here are the ten recommendations for cancer prevention:

- Avoid obesity. Overweight people are more likely to get several types of cancer (They are also more likely to get heart disease and diabetes.) For overweight people, weight loss is protection against disease. Your doctor can help you find the weight loss program that works best for you.
- Cut down on total fat intake. Fats should not exceed thirty percent of your diet. Eating a high-fat diet plays an important part in the incidence of breast, colon and prostrate cancer. This is an effective way to reduce total calories as well.
- Increase the amount and variety of vegetables and fruit in your diet. Vegetables and fruits contain Beta-carotene, Vitamin C, and roughage that reduce your chances of stomach, colon and lung cancer.
- Eat high fiber foods, such as whole grain cereals, vegetables, and fruits. Such foods help move waste products from your colon.
- Limit consumption of alcohol. Heavy drinkers are at a higher risk of cancers of the mouth, throat, and liver.

- Avoid smoked, pickled, or nitrate-cured foods. Eating a lot of ham and chemically cured foods can mean a much higher risk of stomach cancer.
- Do not smoke or chew tobacco.
- Teach yourself, and your daughters as they reach adolescence, to check for lumps in the breast and have a mammogram every two years if you are over forty or have a family history of breast cancer.
- Women should get a Pap smear annually.
- Have your doctor check your stool for blood.

While prevention is best, early detection and treatment can mean a complete cure.

86. FACTS ABOUT CERVICAL CANCER

Let no man deceive himself. If any man among you seemeth to be wise in this world, let him become a fool, that he may be wise.

⁂ 1 Corinthians 3:18

Every woman with a uterus has a cervix. The cervix is the portion of the uterus which is exposed in the vagina and receives the trauma from sexual intercourse and birth. Cervical cancer develops in the lining of the cervix and the good news is that cervical cancer, if it develops, usually develops over a long time. Normal cervical cells may gradually undergo changes to become **precancerous** and then **cancerous**. If you catch the cervical changes in the precancerous stage, cervical cancer is completely treatable! Cervical Intraepithelial Neoplasia (**CIN**) is the term used to describe these abnormal changes. CIN is classified according to the degree of cell abnormality. Low-grade CIN indicates a minimal change in the cells and high-grade CIN indicates a greater degree of abnormality.

Most (80–90 percent) invasive cervical cancer develops in the flat, scaly surface cells that line the cervix (called squamous cell carcinomas). Approximately 10–15 percent of cases develop in glandular surface cells (called adenocarcinomas). Cancer of the cervix is the second most common cancer in women worldwide and is a leading cause of cancer-related death in women in underdeveloped countries. Worldwide, approximately 500,000 cases of cervical cancer are diagnosed each year.

Routine screening has decreased the incidence of invasive cervical cancer in the United States, where approximately 13,000 cases of invasive cervical cancer and 50,000 cases of cervical carcinoma in situ (i.e., localized cancer) are diagnosed yearly. This routine screening is called the Pap test and is a test women should get at least yearly, and some women should get every six months.

Invasive cervical cancer is more common in middle-aged and older women and in women of poor socio-economic status, who are less likely to receive regular screening and early treatment. There is also a higher rate of incidence among African-American, Hispanic, and Native American women.

Sexual activity that increases the risk for infection with HPV and HIV and for cervical cancer includes the following:

- Having multiple sexual partners or having sex with a promiscuous partner
- History of sexually transmitted disease (STD)
- Sexual intercourse at a young age

Women who smoke cigarettes are twice as likely to develop cervical cancer. Chemicals in cigarette smoke may increase the risk by damaging cervical cells.

Other risk factors include age (the condition is rare in women younger than age 15) and race (invasive cancer rates are higher in African Americans, Hispanics, and Native Americans).

Again, the good news is that no woman has to develop or die from cervical cancer because if it is caught early, surgery can eliminate the cancer. Regular screening with a Pap Test effectively lowers the risk for developing invasive cervical cancer by detecting precancerous changes in cervical cells. Women who do not receive regular Pap smears have a higher risk for the condition to develop into invasive cancer.

If the cancer has spread and is invasive treatment includes hysterectomy, radiation and chemotherapy. Cervical cancer should never get to this stage because with the Pap test you and your physician can treat this cancer effectively in the early stages. Also, the best treatment is prevention so if you are not in a monogamous relationship and are sexually active, use condoms.

87. WHAT IS A PAP TEST?

*And they that be wise shall shine as the brightness of the firmament; and
they that turn many to righteousness as the stars for ever and ever.*

ᐁ Daniel 12:3

Diagnosis of cervical cancer includes a Papanicolaou test (Pap
smear) and pelvic examination. The American Cancer Society recommends that all women begin having annual Pap smears at the age
of 18, or when they become sexually active. After three consecutive
negative tests, health care practitioners may perform the test less
often (e.g., every two or three years). The American College of
Obstetrics and Gynecology recommends a yearly Pap smear for all
women who are sexually active. If you have a questionable Pap test,
a positive Pap test or are in a high risk category you may require a
Pap test as often as every six months. Sexual activity that increases
the risk for infection with HPV and HIV and for cervical cancer
includes the following:

- Having multiple sexual partners or having sex with a promiscu-
  ous partner
- History of sexually transmitted disease (STD)
- Sexual intercourse at a young age

In a Pap smear, the health care practitioner removes cells from the
surface of the cervix using a spatula, cotton swab, or brush. The
cells are placed on a glass slide for microscopic evaluation in a laboratory. For accurate results, the test should be performed two
weeks after the end of a menstrual period and at least 48 hours after
sexual intercourse.

Some health care practitioners will confirm the presence of cervical lesions with a colposcopy. After the Pap smear is performed, the
cervix is washed with a diluted vinegar solution and examined for
abnormalities using a light and a magnifying device (a colposcope).
If abnormal areas are detected, further evaluation is necessary,

regardless of the results of the Pap smear. A colposcopy takes a few minutes to perform but may not be covered by insurance.

In a pelvic examination, the vagina and adjacent organs are examined visually and bimanually (using both hands) by your doctor. Visual examination is performed using a speculum (an instrument that is warmed and used to separate the vaginal walls) inserted into the vagina. Next, the organs are palpated (felt with the fingers) by inserting gloved fingers of one hand into the vagina and placing the other hand on the abdomen.

The exam cannot occur until you have the Pap test and pelvic exam. Take control of you destiny and get your annual Pap test.

88. THE STATE OF PROSTATE CANCER

For I would not, brethren, that ye should be ignorant of this mystery, lest ye should be wise in your own conceits;

                                        ᘒ Romans 11:25

Every man is born with a prostate. The prostate produces the hormones needed for sexual activity and for reproduction. The prostate is a gland and prostate cancer is the growth of malignant, fast growing cells in the prostate. The cancer cells reproduce and may spread beyond the prostate gland. The prostate gland sits between a man's bladder and rectum at the bottom of his pelvis. It is about the size of a walnut. Its purpose is to provide sperm with nutrients and protection. Prostate cancer is the growth of malignant cells in the prostate. The cells reproduce and may spread beyond the prostate gland.

Researchers estimate that 50 percent of men over 50 years of age, and 70 percent of men over 70 years of age have some form of prostate cancer. In 2003, in the U.S. alone doctors diagnosed about 220,000 men with prostate cancer and nearly 30,000 men die from prostate cancer each year. Prostate cancer is the second most prevalent cancer among men. African-American men and individuals who have fathers or brothers with prostate cancer appear to be more likely to get the disease.

Most prostate cancer will grow slowly. However, in some cases, prostate cancer can grow rapidly in both younger and older men and become life threatening. If it is not treated, the cancer may spread beyond the prostate gland and reach surrounding tissue and other organs, eventually spreading to other parts of the body.

The good news is that men at risk for developing prostate cancer can catch it early. Just like women should get a yearly Pap test, men should get their prostate checked every year. Your doctor can manually check your prostate by going through your rectum and feeling your prostate with a finger. If this exam is done yearly, any changes in the size or feel of your prostate can be detected and more extensive tests can be done to determine whether you have developed prostate cancer.

The common symptoms of prostate cancer don't always mean the presence of the disease. However, a man who experiences one or more of the following symptoms, particularly if he is at higher risk for prostate cancer, should see his doctor:

- A need to frequently urinate, especially at night
- Difficulty starting urination or holding back urine
- Inability to urinate
- Weak or interrupted urine flow
- Painful or burning urination
- Difficulty obtaining an erection
- Painful ejaculation
- Blood in urine or semen
- Frequent pain or stiffness in the lower back, hips or upper thighs

A variety of conditions may cause these symptoms. For example, as a man ages, his prostate may grow. An enlarged prostate, called benign prostatic hyperplasia (BPH), can block the flow of urine or interfere with sexual function. BPH is not prostate cancer, but can cause many of the same symptoms.

Only a doctor using appropriate tests can determine if a man has prostate cancer, BPH, or another condition with similar symptoms.

There are four major tests for prostate cancer, including the well-known PSA test. These tests fall into two categories: those that screen for the disease, and those that help the doctor determine the stage of the disease when it is found. Screening tests for prostate cancer include:

- **Prostate-specific antigen test (PSA test.)** The PSA test analyzes a blood sample drawn. It checks the sample for PSA, a substance the prostate gland naturally produces to help liquefy semen. A small amount of PSA naturally enters the bloodstream. If higher-than-normal levels of PSA occur (above a level of four mg/ml), it may indicate prostate infection,

inflammation (prostatitis), enlargement of the prostate gland—
or cancer.

- **Digital rectal exam (DRE)**. The prostate is located next to the
  rectum. A doctor performs a digital rectal exam by inserting a
  gloved, lubricated finger into the rectum to examine the
  prostate. If the doctor finds any abnormalities in the texture,
  shape or size of the gland, more tests may be needed.
- **Urine test**. A urine test checks the urine for abnormalities that
  may indicate a problem. The test does not detect prostate cancer, but it can help detect or rule out other conditions with
  similar symptoms.
- **Transrectal ultrasound**. If the doctor has concerns, he or she
  may use transrectal ultrasound to further evaluate the prostate.
  This involves inserting a small probe into the rectum. The
  probe emits sound waves to produce a picture of the prostate
  gland.

Perform a death-defying act! Get your prostate checked!

89. BREAST CANCER—BE A SURVIVOR

Hear instruction, and be wise, and refuse it not.

ఌ Proverbs 8:33

Breast Self Exams should be done regularly so that women at risk for developing breast cancer can catch it early and get definitive treatment in the early stages of breast cancer. The good news for women who develop breast cancer is that in recent years, there's been an explosion of life-saving treatment advances against breast cancer, bringing new hope and excitement. Instead of only one or two options, today there's an overwhelming menu of treatment choices that fight the complex mix of cells in each individual cancer. The decisions—surgery, then perhaps radiation, hormonal (anti-estrogen) therapy, and/or chemotherapy—can feel overwhelming, however, there are many organizations that you and your doctor can tap into that will help you make the best decision for you, for your type of cancer and for your family. There are many breast cancer survivors that can provide helpful and supportive information as you are taking control of both the cancer and your treatment options.

Women with breast cancer have to face many decisions:

- Should they have their breasts removed? Just the one with the cancer or both?
- Should they have radiation therapy or chemotherapy or both?
- Should they have surgery, radiation or chemotherapy or a combination of all three?
- When should they have breast reconstruction?

The best treatment option for you will depend on the type of cancer you have. Before any decisions for treatment are made, you will have a biopsy of the breast lump, which will "STAGE" you breast cancer disease. Once you know the type of cancer you have, do some research on the Internet and read about the options available to you. Talk over the options with your physicians and those that are significant to you and then move deliberately to start your therapy options. What we also know is that breast cancer seems to respond better to treatment if you keep a positive outlook on your life and future—think positively so that your immune system can be at its peak to help you fight the cancer cells. Surgery, radiation and chemotherapy can only eliminate the tumor cells that the treatment can find. Your body's immune system has to do the rest. Your immune system works best when you are rested, in a positive state of mind, have a good nutritional balance and are looking forward to a bright future. You can survive this disease—just talk to the women you know who have had it!

90. COLON CANCER

*And whatsoever hath not fins and scales ye may not eat; it is unclean
unto you.*

ତ୍ତଚ Deuteronomy 14:10

You are born with a colon and both the colon and rectum are important for your nutrition. The colon and rectum are part of the digestive tract. Together, they comprise the large intestine, or large bowel,
which is located in the abdomen between the small intestine and
the anus. Cancer that originates in the colon or rectum is called colorectal cancer.

The colon absorbs water, electrolytes, and nutrients from food
and transports them into the bloodstream. It is about six feet in
length and consists of the cecum (connects to the small intestine at
the cecal valve), the ascending colon (the vertical segment located
on the right side of the abdomen), the transverse colon (extends
across the abdomen), the descending colon (leads vertically down
the left side of the abdomen), and the sigmoid colon (extends to the
rectum).

The rectum is the last segment of the large intestine. It is 8 to 10
inches in length and leads to the anus, which is the opening to the
outside of the body. Waste material (fecal matter) is stored in the rectum until it is eliminated from the body through the anus.

Most (over 95 percent) colorectal cancers are **adenocarcinomas** that develop when a change (i.e., mutation) occurs in cells that
line the wall of the colon or rectum. The disease often begins as an
intestinal **polyp**, also called an adenoma, which is an abnormal
growth of tissue. Polyps gradually can become precancerous and
then cancerous.

Incidence of colorectal cancer is highest in developed countries
such as the United States and Japan, and lowest in developing countries in Africa and Asia. It is the third most common type of cancer
in both men and women in the United States. Incidence are slightly

higher in men than women, and is highest in African-American men.

The American Cancer Society estimates that about 145,000 cases of colorectal cancer will be diagnosed and about 56,000 people will die from the disease in 2005. The death rate from colorectal cancer has declined over the past 15 years due to improved screening methods and advances in treatment.

Colorectal cancer can be asymptomatic (i.e., it may not cause symptoms). **Blood in the stool** is a common sign of the disease. Blood may be bright red or dark in color, and may not be noticeable. Chronic bleeding may result in iron deficiency **anemia**, which may cause fatigue and pale skin.

Other symptoms include the following:

- Abdominal discomfort (e.g., pain, bloating, cramping, fullness)
- Change in bowel habits
- Constipation or diarrhea
- Narrow stools
- Nausea and vomiting
- Unexplained weight loss

Diagnosis involves **screening** to detect colorectal cancer in asymptomatic patients (i.e., those without symptoms) with no family history of the disease. Screening is recommended beginning at age 50 and includes the following:

- Digital rectal examination (DRE) and fecal occult blood test annually and
- Double-contrast barium enema every five to ten years and
- Flexible sigmoidoscopy every five years, or
- Total colonoscopy every ten years

Diagnosis of colorectal cancer in symptomatic patients and high-risk patients includes laboratory and imaging tests. **Biopsy** (i.e., removal of a tissue sample for examination under a microscope) is necessary to confirm the diagnosis.

In a **digital rectal examination** (DRE), the physician inserts a lubricated, gloved finger into the patient's rectum to feel for tumors.

Approximately 5–10 percent of colorectal cancers are palpable (i.e., able to be felt).

Fecal occult blood test is used to detect microscopic blood in the stool, which may indicate early colorectal cancer. When results of this test are positive, the diagnosis is confirmed using additional procedures (e.g., barium enema, sigmoidoscopy, colonoscopy).

When colorectal cancer is suspected, **laboratory tests** such as urinalysis, blood tests (e.g., carcinoembryonic antigen level, complete blood count, electrolyte and chemical panels), and imaging tests are performed.

Staging is a method of evaluating the progress of the cancer in a patient. That is, it looks at the tumor and the extent to which it has spread to other parts of the body. Once doctors know how far along the cancer is, they can decide on the best course of treatment.

Surgery is the treatment of choice for colorectal cancer. Treatment depends on the *stage* of the disease and the overall health of the patient. Chemotherapy and radiation therapy may be used as adjuvant treatment (i.e., in addition to surgery).

SECTION IX

TAKE A MINUTE FOR YOUR LUNGS

91. BREATHING EASIER DURING ALLERGY SEASON

The God who made the world and everything in it; being Lord of heaven and earth, does not live in shrines made by man, nor is he served by human hands, as though he needed anything, since he himself gives to all man life and breath and everything.

ᕤ Acts 17: 24–5

If it's late fall or early spring, it's sneezing time again. But allergy season doesn't have to be as bad as last year. This time, you will know how to help yourself feel better.

An *allergy* is an over-reaction that happens when your body desperately tries to get rid of something you breathed in, such as ragweed or other pollen; or something you ate; or even something you touched, such as poison ivy. Your body reacts to these invaders with symptoms such as headaches, itchy eyes, sneezing, coughing, and skin rashes.

Here are some useful tips about allergies:

- Avoid the things that can trigger your allergies. If you do not know what these are, get tested. Your doctor or health clinic can refer you to someone who can do the tests.
- If you can't avoid the irritant that triggers your allergy, take antihistamines (Benadryl™, Allerest™, Contac™, Chlortrimiton™, etc.) as directed by your doctor,
- Use an air-conditioner and air cleaner in your home. (But keep in mind, if the temperature gets lower than 700, it can trigger sneezing. This is often mistaken as a "cold."
- If you have a window air conditioning unit, leave the unit off when it is not needed.
- Bright light may trigger sneezing, so wear sunglasses.
- Alcohol can make you more sensitive to allergens (the irritants that trigger the reaction). So, turning down a drink may also turn down your allergies.

- Take allergy medicines before you go to bed, in order to avoid feeling sluggish during the day.
- Don't use Kleenex or paper products to blow your nose–you may be allergic to the paper dust. It is better to use handkerchiefs, but be careful about the detergents and bleaches you use, since you may be allergic to these as well. Double rinsing helps get such ingredients out of your clothes.
- Put a plastic covering over your old mattress or stuffed chair, especially if it has animal fur or feathers, and keep your living environment clean.
- Avoid foods like watermelon, avocados, mangos, or tropical drinks that may make your mouth and throat itch.

In the old days, people with allergies moved to desert climates, where there was less pollen to cause allergies. But today, southwestern states like Arizona are no safer than anywhere else. What happened is that the people who moved there to avoid pollens and grasses ended up putting in golf courses, nice lawns, flowers, and trees. Yes, people can be funny.

92. LIVING WITH ASTHMA

I prophesied as he commanded me, and the breath came into them, and they lived, and stood upon their feet, an exceedingly great host."

ఞ Ezekiel 37:10

Asthma is a disease of the airways in your lungs. About five percent of children suffer from asthma, and this rate is increasing. The rate among Latino children under 18 is 7.8 percent; for African-American children, 4.2 percent; and for White children, 2.9 percent. The number of children from the inner city who die from asthma has doubled in the last ten years.

Asthma leads to more visits to emergency rooms and absences from school than any other childhood illness. When an asthma attack occurs, the small airways in the lungs close up, plugged with mucous. This blocking of air usually produces a lot of wheezing and coughing, and, in some cases, life-or-death struggle for oxygen that may last a few minutes but can go on for weeks. Even a short asthma attack can be a frightening experience.

If you or someone you know is prone to get asthma attacks, prevention is better than cure. In this case, this means, you can minimize attacks by learning to identify and avoid irritants like dust and smoke or pollens, or animal dander. If your house is in a neighborhood where the air is especially bad, you may want to get an air filter. And be sure your furnace filters get changed when they're dirty. Do this for yourself, your children, and your family.

Asthma doesn't have to be a disabling illness. Asthma patients play professional sports, win gold medals at the Olympic games, become successful politicians and scientists, and live very normal lives. The trick is to take the good drugs available to help clear the lungs and airways. Talk to your doctor about them.

The asthma patient can also help her-or-himself by:

- Not smoking or allowing others to smoke around them
- Exercising regularly

- Keeping an inhaler within reach at all times
- Warming up properly before exercise
- Avoiding things that may cause allergic reactions such as cats, dogs, smoke, and dust, pollens, etc.
- Staying indoors during air pollution alerts
- Not becoming over-excited and keeping anger in check
- Not using asthma as an excuse to get sympathy or for not doing things you could but don't want to do.
- Eating sensibly, learning to recognize foods that may bring on an attack, and avoiding fat in your diet

Reading and learning as much as you can about the disease, because the more you know, the better able you are to handle problems that may arise.

93. THE COMMON COLD

And they that shall be of thee shall build the old waste places: thou shalt raise up the foundations of many generations; and thou shalt be called, The repairer of the breach, The restorer of paths to dwell in.

            ∾ Isaiah 58:12

The average person catches two colds per year. Colds are caused not by one but by about two hundred viruses grouped together. A cold starts when a virus penetrates the cells of your lungs and surrounding tissue. By the time you begin to experience a sore throat, runny nose, and headache, you may have already had the cold for several days.

The reason you tend to catch more colds in winter is that the dry indoor air dries out your mucous membranes and lowers your resistance to viruses. We often catch colds from one another. If you touch the hand of someone with a cold and then touch your own nose, you're likely to catch the cold. Inhaling droplets from someone sneezing near you can also infect you. A sneeze has about 5,000 droplets and can travel across a crowded room for up to twelve feet

We know that you can't catch a cold from sitting in a draft, or being exposed to cold temperatures, night air, the rain, or any combination of hot and cold temperatures. You can go out into the cold air immediately after a hot bath without catching a cold. Your child won't catch a cold just by going out into the chill of winter without a coat, even if he was sweating from exercise or heat. He may sneeze from an allergic reaction if he gets his feet in cold water, but he can't catch a cold from not wearing his boots.

As you get older, you are likely to get fewer and fewer colds. Older people develop immunity from previous colds. They are also more careful about germs, so they wash their hands regularly. Babies can get a cold almost every month. Teenagers get about three colds per year. As young people become parents, they will again get frequent colds from their children.

The best way to avoid colds is to eat a healthy diet and take care of your general health, so that your body will be strong enough to fight the virus. Wash your hands three times a day. Get enough sleep. When you become overly tired, you become vulnerable.

If you go to the doctor and take cold remedies, it will take a week to recover. If you do nothing, it will take seven days. There is no cure for the common cold. Cold remedies treat only the symptoms. For instance, anti-histamines will stop only your sneezing and itching eyes.

Should you feed a cold and starve a fever? Actually, you should feed both, even when you don't feel like eating. Any kind of infection will sap your energy, so you need to replenish your calories to keep up your strength. It's actually true that chicken soup is a good food for a cold. It feels good going down and the steam opens your clogged nose.

While you are sick, get plenty of rest, keep warm, drink plenty of fluids, and eat easily digestible foods.

SECTION X

———◦∿◦———

TAKE A MINUTE TO LEARN ABOUT COMMON MEDICAL PROBLEMS

94. ANEMIA

We then that are strong ought to bear the infirmities of the weak, and not to please ourselves.

ᕙᕗ Romans 15:1

Your body is composed of cells that need oxygen to do their job. If the cells that transfer oxygen are in poor condition or there are not enough of them to deliver what your body needs, you have what people call "iron poor blood," "low blood count"—or simply *anemia.*

Anemia causes lethargy, dizziness, tiredness and headaches. It occurs when the red blood cells in your body are being destroyed more quickly than they are being made. This can happen because you are not eating the right foods, you are bleeding internally, or your body is unable to make enough red blood cells.

If you have anemia symptoms, consult your doctor. You can also help yourself by eating right. Foods high in the iron and vitamin B12 your blood needs including:

- Fruit
- Whole grain breads
- Beans
- Lean meats
- Fish
- Green vegetables.

People often get low blood pressure and low blood count confused. There is no disease called "low blood pressure." Generally, the lower your blood pressures, the better off you are, if you are not bleeding nor have some other health problem.

Blood pressure describes the amount of pressure in your blood. *Anemia* (or low blood count) refers to the quantity of red blood cells in your blood.

Women should get their red blood cells count checked each year when they get a Pap smear. So should anyone with black stool or who has been spitting up blood.

Remember, there is power in the blood.

95. STOMACH PAIN

Do you not know that your body is a temple of the Holy Spirit who is in you, whom you have from God, and that you are not your own? For you have been bought with a price: therefore, glorify God in your body.

           ໑ 1 Corinthians 6:19–20

Everybody has a painful stomach now and then, because of gas caused by overeating, eating spicy food, drinking alcohol, or just being upset. Stomach pain often goes along with belching, nausea, vomiting, rumbling noises, gas, diarrhea, or constipation. Most of the time it goes away with the help of a little Pepto-Bismol, Rolaids, mint tea, or other antacids, activated charcoal, or the use of a heating pad.

But under certain conditions the pain could be a sign of stomach ulcers, kidney disorders, a urinary infection, appendicitis, hernia, or food poisoning. Here are red light warning systems to watch for:

- Severe pain
- Pain that doesn't go away after home remedy
- Pain accompanied by a fever
- Diarrhea
- A burning sensation when you urinate
- Vomiting blood
- Feeling weak

Bacteria such as E-Coli or Salmonella, which we can be exposed to if we eat contaminated foods, are the cause of most food poisoning. Both can be present in raw eggs, improperly handled meats, dairy products, seafood, and poultry. Food handlers who do not wash their hands after going to the toilet can also transmit E-Coli to food.

E-coli and Salmonella take twelve-to twenty-four hours before they produce symptoms of stomach pain, vomiting, diarrhea, fever and chill. Such infections usually last for two to three days and are rarely fatal, but it *can* be fatal to the very young and very old. Each year about five hundred infants and old people die from diseases caused by food-borne bacteria.

You can protect yourself by washing with soap and very hot water pots and pans and plates in which you've put raw meats. Thoroughly cook eggs, fish, and chicken before eating them.

Food poisoning can spoil a picnic. Avoid eggs, salad dressing, and dairy products at picnics if they can't be kept cold. Keep hot foods hot and cold foods cold.

Most cases of food poisoning can be treated with bed rest and plenty of mint tea, activated charcoal tablets, fruit juices, and broth. More serious or persistent cases should be treated by a physician.

96. LIVING WITH ARTHRITIS

And he said unto him, Arise, go thy way: thy faith hath made thee whole.

ᏂᎤ Luke 17:19

Arthritis causes more crippling and discomfort than any other chronic disease and affects about 43 million Americans, or one in six of us, of all ages. Every family has elderly members, especially women, who suffer from some form of arthritis. The chief complaints are likely to be about the aching, pain, stiffness, swelling, and tenderness brought on by joint motion.

The most common type of arthritis is osteoarthritis. It results from damage to the ligaments and coverings of the joints in the hands, feet, knees, elbows, ankles and spine. The chief cause is years and years of wear and tear on these joints. That is why it is referred to as "gray hair of the joints." Other causes include injury, hormonal changes, and heredity.

Don't believe the old myths that arthritis patients should not exercise. Aerobic exercise actually reduces joint pain, increases strength and also improves disposition. Try walking, dancing, swimming or bicycling. Be sure to rest your joints, however, if they should become painful.

Surgery is sometimes recommended in severe cases of arthritis to prevent deformities and restore joint function in knees, hips, and shoulders. But for most people, a heating pad, massage, aspirin, and other medication will help. There are a number of splints, braces, and corsets that can give relief. If you are overweight, losing weight will be a great favor to your joints.

Arthritis can't be cured, but with appropriate medical care, pain and discomfort can be reduced. Research suggests that doxycline, an antibiotic commonly used in treatment for acne, blocks enzymes in the joint that damage the cartilage. Another antibiotic, minocycline, may offer some relief. Glucosamine and chondroitin have been touted in the best seller, *The Arthritis Cure*. Other new arthritis treatments on the way include Hyaluronic acid, Enbrel, and Arava (a new drug therapy).

97. LIVING WITH EPILEPSY AND SEIZURES

Therefore seeing we have this ministry, as we have received mercy, we faint not. . . .

                 ❧ 2 Corinthians 4:1

Epilepsy is the medical term for convulsions, seizures or fits. It is caused by uncontrolled, involuntary activity in the brain. Typically, a person having a seizure has jerky arm and leg movements, does not respond when spoken to, and, most importantly, does not remember having the seizure. Not all seizures involve jerky movements; some seizures just cause the person to stare off into space. But in both cases, the person will not remember having had a seizure.

Epilepsy can be with you at birth or can be caused by drugs, alcohol, tumors, injuries or diseases of the brain. Seizures can be prevented by medications. But most of these medications have side effects of which patients should be aware.

Treatment of children raises a special problem. Sometimes children are prescribed Phenobarbital to control seizures. Phenobarbital can reduce the child's attention span and short-term memory. But, when the drug is withdrawn, the child usually regains short-term memory, and whatever negative effects it may have had on his or her ability to think will reverse.

The two most common types of epilepsy attacks are:

- *Petit Mal* (little attacks), which usually occur in childhood and stop before twenty years of age. These attacks are characterized by brief periods of inattentiveness or even unconsciousness. These attacks can occur up to 100 times per day and may or may not be followed by Grand Mal seizures.
- *Grand Mal* is more common and dramatic. The patient usually loses consciousness and falls, which may result in injury. The patient may also bite their tongue and lose bladder and bowel control. After the attack, the patient usually falls asleep

or feels confused and disoriented. Pain in the stomach and head may follow.

Both children and adults with epilepsy can live normally. Children can do very well at school, and adults can find employment. But children at school and adults on the workplace should select activities or jobs that don't place them around fire, water, machinery, or heights.

To prevent seizures from occurring, patients should take their medication as prescribed, get enough sleep, avoid alcohol, and not go for long periods without food.

If you are trying to help someone who has a seizure, place a padded gag between the patient's teeth to keep the airway open and to prevent him or her from biting their tongue. It is also a good idea to restrain the patient to reduce the risk of injury.

Since biblical times, there have been myths and superstitions about epilepsy. But in fact there is no danger in being around a person prone to epileptic seizures. Most people with epilepsy live normal healthy lives if they take their medication as prescribed.

98. DRY EYES

In whom the God of this world hath blinded the minds of them which believe not, lest he light of the glorious gospel of Christ, who is the image of God, should shine unto them.

☥ *2 Corinthians 4:4*

Your eyes are called the windows to your soul, but those windows can get dry and irritated, bloodshot and red, as the result of hay fever, dust, smoke, or foreign particles. Most such irritations are minor, but they can sometimes damage your eyes' delicate tissue. Dryness of the eyes can even cause loss of sight.

Over nine million people describe their eyes as feeling blurry and gritty. Whether you are one of them depends on whether your eyes produce many tears. (So tears are good for the body, as well as the soul.) Some people produce many tears, some do not. The fewer tears you produce, the more irritation you are likely to have.

Older people are more likely to have dry eyes because the tear glands slow down as we age. Being female also puts you at higher risk. Living in dry climates can mean trouble too. People who live in Arizona, or other hot, arid climates can brag about their year-round sunshine, but they also have more problems with dry eyes.

Even the way we heat and cool our indoor air can make a difference. Low moisture indoor heating may cause eye irritation. So may air conditioning. In fact, any dry air or wind will tend to dry out your eyes.

Stress plays a role here too. The intense concentration that stress brings about causes us to blink less often, so we tend to have dry eyes in times of stress. Also, when eyelids don't close properly, as in patients with Bell's palsy, dry eyes can be a problem. Dry eyes can also be a side effect of medications like diuretics, antihistamines, beta-blockers, decongestants, birth control pills, and sleeping pills.

You can treat dry eyes with tear replacement drops. There are over thirty types on the market. Experiment to see which one works best for you. One drop in each eye every three hours, whether the eyes feel dry or not, will help. Using such drops can be a preventive act.

Don't use these drops more than five times per day. If you use them too often, the preservative can build up toxins that can damage the surface of the eye. The preservative-free compounds are "Refresh™" and "Ocu-Tears™." *Don't use anti-redness drops that constrict the blood vessels. They are not the same as tear replacement drops.*

Other options are moisture chamber glasses, humidifiers, and even surgery. If the problem persists, talk to your doctor about it, especially if you wear contact lenses.

99. WHAT TO TAKE WITH YOU WHEN YOU TRAVEL

When thou passeth through the waters, I will be with thee; and through the rivers, they shall not overflow thee: when thou walkest through the fire, thou shalt not be burned; neither shall the flame kindle upon thee.

                                                ☙ Isaiah 43:2

Sometimes, health problems come up while we're traveling. By doing a little planning ahead, you can avoid some health problems, and be sure that you're ready to deal with any health problem that does come up for you and your family. Just follow these steps:

- Be sure you will not run out of your prescription medicines.
- Drink plenty of fluids and exercise often to keep your energy up.
- Travel can be hard on your stomach. If you're traveling abroad, you'll be eating new foods and going through the stresses of customs and security. So take along some antacids—for heartburn, upset stomach, and indigestion.
- Anti-diarrhea medications or activated charcoal tablets can soothe your stomach, by stopping the cramping, and diarrhea in cases of food poisoning.
- Laxatives can also come in handy. Children sometimes need them. Just eating in a strange place can cause constipation. Kids sometimes go to camp for a week and return home without having made a bowel movement all week.
- Antibiotic cream or an antiseptic can help keep little cuts and bruises from becoming infected.
- An anti-itch cream can help relieve itching caused by insect bites, poison ivy, and rashes.
- Aspirins or other analgesics come in handy for toothaches, muscle aches, menstrual cramps, arthritis pain, strains, inflammation, and fever.

- Decongestants relieve nasal congestion and can prevent earaches caused by fluid buildup in high altitudes.
- Moisturizing cream can help work against the sun and wind, which can dry out your skin. You'll probably be out doors a lot when you travel, so use sunscreen too. It protects your skin against the damaging effects of ultraviolet light.
- Eye drops soothe and protect dry, scratchy eyes.
- An extra pair of eyeglasses is handy in case your regular pair is lost or stolen.
- If you are prone to get motion sickness, take antihistamines. Don't read while in motion, and sit on the left side of planes. Airplanes bank to the right more than they bank to the left.
- Make sure you have health coverage where you are away.

100. WHO SHOULD GET A FLU SHOT?

When you eat of the fruit of your own hands, you will be happy and it will be well with you.

ಅ Psalms 128:2

The flu, caused by a virus, can make you feel really bad. You're hot one minute, cold the next, your headaches, and your energy is gone. Some people never get the flu whether they get the flu shot or not. Others swear by flu shots. Talk to your doctor about your best option.

What Is the Flu Shot?

The flu shot is a vaccine that protects against the influenza virus. Like other shots you've had it helps your body fight infections. The flu shot contains a small amount of dead flu virus. The flu shot won't give you the flu, but those dead viruses are enough to get your body's immune system ready to fight off the real flu when it comes around next winter.

Who Should Get the Flu Shot?

Almost anyone can get a flu shot, but most kids who are healthy don't need it, because even if they get the flu, they'll probably just be sick for a little while and then get better. But there are some kids who may get very sick if they catch the flu, so doctors recommend that these kids get the flu shot. Kids who have asthma or other lung problems, heart problems, kidney disease, diabetes or sickle cell anemia should get the flu shot every year. Check with your doctor.

Another reason to get a flu shot is to protect someone in your family who might get very sick if that person caught the flu from you. If you live with someone who has any of the medical problems listed above and you get the flu that person could get very sick. Older people also should get the flu shot because their immune system (the body's disease fighting system) isn't as strong as a younger, healthy person.

Babies and little kids can get very sick from the flu and doctors encourage parents to have their kids who are between six months and two years-old to get a flu shot. Babies younger than six months of age can get sick from the shot itself and they are not in the age group where a shot is recommended. If you have questions regarding the age your child should be to get a flu shot ask your doctor.

A yearly flu shot is recommended for the following groups of people who are at increased risk from serious complications from the flu:

- People ages 50 years and older
- residents of nursing homes and other long-term care facilities that house people of any age who have long-term illnesses.
- Adults and children six months of age or older who have either a chronic heart or lung disease such as asthma or cystic fibrosis.
- Adults and children six months of age or older who need regular medical care or had to be in a hospital because of metabolic diseases, like diabetes, chronic kidney disease, or weakened immune system, including immune system problems caused by medicine or by infection with HIV.
- Children and teenagers aged six months to 18 years who are on long-term aspirin therapy and therefore could develop Reye's Syndrome after the flu.
- Women who are more than three months pregnant during the flu season.

If you or your family member fits one of the situations listed above you may benefit from the flu shot.

101. WHAT IS SLEEP APNEA?

In any case thou shall deliver him the pledge again when the sun goes down, that he may sleep in his own raiment and bless thee; and it shall be righteousness unto thee before the Lord thy God.

                 ᏔᏮ Deuteronomy 24:13

Sleep apnea happens when you stop breathing during sleep. There are three types of sleep apnea: obstructive sleep apnea, central sleep apnea and a combination of the two called mixed sleep apnea. Obstructive sleep apnea (OSA) is the most common and is caused by a blockage of the airway by the back of the throat. When you sleep, the soft tissue in the rear of the throat collapses and closes and when that happens it blocks your windpipe. In central sleep apnea, the airway is not blocked but the brain fails to signal the muscles to breathe. Mixed apnea, as the name implies, is a combination of the two. With each apnea event, the brain briefly arouses people with sleep apnea in order for them to resume breathing, but consequently sleep is extremely fragmented and of poor quality. Also, during the time you have apnea, the brain, heart and other organs are not getting the oxygen it needs. Your brain cannot function with oxygen so it is important to have your sleep apnea treated.

Sleep apnea is very common-as common as adult diabetes-and affects more than twelve million Americans, according to the National Institutes of Health. Risk factors include being male, overweight, and over the age of 40, but sleep apnea can strike anyone at any age, even children. Yet, because of the lack of awareness by the public and healthcare professionals, the vast majority remain undiagnosed and therefore untreated, despite the fact that this serious disorder can have significant consequences.

Untreated, sleep apnea can cause high blood pressure and other cardiovascular diseases because a lack of oxygen can strain the heart, specifically the right side of the heart. Because you don't sleep well, sleep apnea can cause memory problems, weight gain, impotency, and headaches. Moreover, untreated sleep apnea may be responsible for job impairment and motor vehicle crashes because you are always tired from a lack of sleep. Fortunately, sleep apnea can be diagnosed and treated. Several treatment options exist, and research into additional options continues.

If you snore a lot and wake yourself up from snoring, you may have sleep apnea. You should ask your doctor whether a sleep apnea study is a good test for you. Also, if your wife tells you that you have "happy feet" or "running feet" when you sleep there is a good chance you have sleep apnea. Don't delay, see your doctor about this problem before you stress your heart out.

102. WHY DO PEOPLE SNORE AND IS IT DANGEROUS?

And Jacob awaked out of his sleep, and he said, Surely the Lord is in this place; and I knew it not.

ᏮᎧ Genesis 28:16

The back of your throat has three structures that work together to produce snoring. The soft palate, the uvula (the little think that hangs down at the back of your throat) and the tonsils. When these three structures flap against each other or if the tonsils block the air passage at the back of your throat, you get snoring.

People who snore have one of the following problems:

- Less than normal muscle tone in the tongue or throat
- A lot of tissue in the back of the throat
- A blocked nasal passage
- A soft palate or uvula that blocks the back of the throat

If the blockage from snoring obstructs the back of the throat, it can lead to sleep apnea which is a serious medical condition. If your snoring wakes you up multiple times during the night or your wife or husband say you have "happy or running" feet you may not just have snoring you may have sleep apnea.

Even though snoring may be an indication of a more serious problem, most of the time you don't have to worry if you snore. Some facts about snoring:

- 20 percent of the population snores
- Males and obese people have more problems with snoring than females and people of average weight
- Snoring will be louder if you are sleeping on your back

Talk to your doctor about your snoring problem and if both you and the doctor think it is serious enough your doctor will order tests for you to rule out sleep apnea.

Pleasant Dreams.

103. WRINKLES AND BOTOX

Thou shalt rise up before the hoary head, and honour the face of the old man, and fear thy God: I [am] the LORD.

၅ Leviticus 19.32

Did you know that one of the easiest ways to tell the age of adults is by looking at their faces, or more specifically, at their skin? As people age, all the time they've spent in the sun, at tanning salons, or smoking cigarettes, catches up with them. The result is often—you guessed it—wrinkles!

The skin is made up of three layers: the **epidermis** (say: eh-pih-**dur**-miss), the dermis, and the **subcutaneous** (say: sub-cyoo-**tay**-nee-us) layer. The outermost layer of the skin that everyone can see is the epidermis, the middle is the dermis, and the innermost layer is the subcutaneous layer. All three work together to keep the skin smooth and beautiful.

When you are young, the skin does a great job of stretching and holding in moisture. The dermis has an elastic quality thanks to fibers called **elastin** that keep the skin looking and feeling young. A protein in the dermis called **collagen** (say: **ka**-le-jen) also plays a part in preventing wrinkles.

However, over time, the dermis loses both collagen and elastin, so skin gets thinner and has trouble getting enough moisture to the epidermis. The fat in the subcutaneous layer that gives skin a plump appearance also begins to disappear, the epidermis starts to sag, and wrinkles form.

There's not a magic age (like 40) where everyone suddenly gets wrinkles. Some people in their 20's have little wrinkles around their eyes (called "crow's feet") from squinting or spending too much time in the sun. Other people may be in their 50's or 60's before you can even see a wrinkle. This is usually because they have taken good care of their skin over the years and may have more **sebum** (say: **see**-bum), the skin's natural oil. They may also have "good genes" - which means their family members don't have many wrinkles either.

I wish I had inherited some of Lena Horne's genes. Eventually, however, everyone will have at least a few wrinkles. It's a natural part of the aging process.

Here are some things people can do to prevent getting many wrinkles at an early age:

Avoid spending too much time in the direct sun, especially during the hours when the sun's rays are harshest (between 10:00 AM and 4:00 PM). Ultraviolet (UV) rays cause many wrinkles. Sunblock helps, but it doesn't block out all the damaging UV rays that cause wrinkles to the skin. Still, if you are outside a lot, be sure to wear a sunblock with sun protection factor (SPF) 15 or higher and reapply often (every two to three hours). Always reapply after swimming or playing sports that make you sweat!

- Don't go to the tanning salon. The UV light from tanning booths is just as damaging as the sun's - and sometimes worse.
- Don't smoke! Smoking robs your skin of precious moisture and causes premature (early) wrinkles. (Did you ever notice that most heavy smokers have wrinkles around their mouths?).
- Moisturize dry skin every day with a hydrating cream or moisturizer, especially during months when the air is drier.
- Drink lots of *water* every day to keep hydrated and help your skin stay moist and smooth.

Now that you have learned that "wrinkles" involve the skin and not muscles tissues let's see if Botox treatments will treat your wrinkles. Botox treatment involves injecting very small amounts of the purified toxin into the wrinkles. This toxin is made from the same bacteria that cause food poisoning or Botulism. Botox is injected into the muscles of your face that produce frown lines—usually the muscles of your forehead and around your nose. Within two or three days, the muscles that produce frown lines lose their ability to contract in order to produce the frown lines by blocking the nerves to those muscles. For the next three months or so after you're treated, you can't frown even if you try. After that, the effect gradually decreases until muscles return to normal about six months after the treatment, at which point the treatment can then be repeated.

Building on their success with frown lines, doctors now use Botox to treat wrinkles around the eyes ("crows' feet"), as well as lines on the forehead and neck.

The effect of Botox is not permanent. The downside of Botox treatment is that it needs repeating every six months or so. The upside is that complications, which don't happen very often, also go away over time. Sometimes, a muscle that has been repeatedly injected eventually loses its ability to contract and doesn't need to be treated anymore. However, this is not an outcome you can count on.

The major complication of Botox is weakening of muscles in the vicinity that you didn't want treated. Improper injection to frown lines, for instance, can result in a temporary eyelid droop. This goes away in the same three to six month period.

Doctors familiar with the proper use of Botox can generally avoid even mild and temporary side effects. It is therefore a good idea to ask around and be sure the dermatologist or plastic surgeon you consult is experienced.

Injection sessions generally cost several hundred dollars, depending on how much work you have done. Insurance rarely covers Botox treatments that are intended for cosmetic improvement.

Whether you use Botox or not is up to you, just know that it will not reverse the affects of aging on your skin. Also aging is a good thing—the alternative is not so good.

104. WHEN DO I NEED AN ANTIBIOTIC?

And Jesus went about all Galilee, teaching in their synagogues, and preaching the gospel of the kingdom, and healing all manner of sickness and all manner of disease among the people.

ॐ Matthew 4:23

Antibiotics are medicines that fight (or prevent) infections that are caused by bacteria. Bacteria are also called germs. If the infection is caused by a virus, antibiotics can't fight the virus. When bacteria are exposed to the same antibiotics, after a while the antibiotic can't fight the germs anymore. Being exposed to the same antibiotic for a long time can make some germs change or mutate. Sometimes germs just change by themselves. Some of the changes make the germs so strong, they can fight back against antibiotics and win the fight. These strong germs can live and multiply, even while you are taking antibiotics. These germs are said to be "resistant" to this antibiotic. Germs can even become resistant to many antibiotics. Antibiotic resistance is becoming a common problem in many parts of the United States. If your infection is resistant to the antibiotic you are taking, your infection can last longer. Instead of getting better, your infection might get worse. You might have to make several visits to your doctor's office. You might have to take different medicines or go to a hospital for antibiotics given intravenously (in your veins).

At the same time, your family members or other people you come in contact with may catch the resistant germs that you have. Then these people might also get infections that are hard to cure. Your doctor will want to prescribe antibiotics only for illnesses that are caused by germs. These illnesses include infections such as strep throat, urinary tract infections and ear infections. People sometimes ask their doctor for antibiotics when they have a viral illness, such as a cold, the flu (influenza) or mononucleosis (mono). Antibiotics cannot cure any viral illnesses.

You should not push your doctor to give you or your children antibiotics for a viral illness. Instead, ask your doctor for things you can do to make you feel better. Every time you take antibiotics when you don't really need them, you increase the chance that you will get an illness someday that is caused by germs that are resistant to antibiotics.

Follow your doctor's directions carefully. Your doctor will tell you to take the entire antibiotic. Don't stop taking your antibiotic just because you feel better. Taking less of an antibiotic when you need it will not help prevent antibiotic resistance.

Wash your hands with soap and water before you eat and after you use the bathroom. Regular hand washing will help keep you healthy and prevent the spread of germs.

Also, ask your doctor if you have all the vaccinations (shots) you need to protect yourself from illness.

105. PEER PRESSURE—PARENTS CAN BE GOOD RELEASE VALVES

And Jesus went about all Galilee, teaching in their synagogues, and preaching the gospel of the kingdom, and healing all manner of sickness and all manner of disease among the people.

ᏗᎥ Matthew 4:23

As your children grow older they will be faced with some challenging decisions. Some decisions don't have a clear 'right' or 'wrong' answer—like, should they play soccer or field hockey? Other decisions involve serious moral questions, like whether to cut class, try alcohol, cigarettes, or drugs, or lie to their parents.

Peer pressure occurs at all ages. However, most adults have learned when to follow the crowd and when to make their own decisions. Making decisions on one's own is hard enough, but when other people get involved and try to pressure you or your children one way or another, it can be even harder. People who are your age, like your friends or classmates, are called peers. When they try to influence how you act, to get you to do something, it's called **peer pressure**. It's something everyone has to deal with—even adults. Let's talk about how to handle it.

Humans are pack animals—we are clannish and work best in numbers as opposed to being isolated. Peers influence your life, even if you don't realize it, just by spending time with you. You learn from them, and they learn from you. It's only human nature to listen to and learn from other people in your age group.

Peers can have a positive influence on each other, whether you learn from them or their mistakes. Maybe a coworker tried solving a problem one way and it had less than an optimal outcome or another student in your child's science class taught him or her an easy way to remember the planets of the solar system, or someone on your bowling league or your son's soccer team taught you a cool trick with the ball. You might admire a friend who is always a good sport and try to be more like him or her. Maybe you got others excited about your new favorite book dance, or music, and now everyone's reading, dancing, or listening to it. These are examples of how peers positively influence each other every day.

Sometimes peers influence each other in negative ways. For example, a few kids in school might try to get your child to cut class with them or experiment with drugs, alcohol or cigarettes. You can't be with your children 24 hours a day and have to let them make their own decisions; it is the process of maturity. Some kids give in to peer pressure because they want to be liked, to fit in, or because they worry that other kids may make fun of them if they don't go along with the group. Others may go along because they are curious to try something new that others are doing. The idea that "everyone's doing it" may influence some kids to leave their better judgment, or their common sense, behind. The issue is to provide your children with a way to say "no" without fear of losing their position in the hierarchy of their world.

It's tough for you and your children to say "no" to peer pressure, but it can be done. Paying attention to your own feelings and beliefs about what is right and wrong can help you know the right thing to do. Inner strength and self-confidence can help you stand firm, walk away, and resist doing something when you know better. It is also helpful for your children to use their parents as excuses to say no — they could always use the excuse that "I'd like to say yes but my parents will kill me." It is also helpful to have your kids see you say no to peer pressure and do the right thing for the right reason, like standing up to prejudice or fighting for the rights of the under privileged. Usually it takes one person to stand up for what's right to start a whole new trend in peer pressure. Take a chance and be a leader.

106. WHAT IS ALZHEIMER'S OR OLD TIMER'S DISEASE?

The glory of young men [is] their strength: and the beauty of old men [is] the gray head.

ை Proverbs 20:29

About four million people in the U.S. have Alzheimer's or "Old Timer's" disease. In the early stages most people affected with Alzheimer's disease just seem to be forgetful or become moody. Alzheimer's disease can last 10 to 20 years during which it becomes harder for the person with the disease to remember, think, and use language. In the mid-to-late stages of the disease the person with Alzheimer's disease may have a hard time with loud noises or with too many people in the room. Their vision is altered—especially depth perception which makes it difficult for them to walk, dress themselves or eat from a plate.

After a while, people with Alzheimer's have a hard time with things like using the phone, dressing, cooking, or managing money. Sadly, many people think the early symptoms of Alzheimer's are signs of normal aging. So Alzheimer's is often not diagnosed and treated early. The disease is more common in older adults. And it affects all races. About one in ten people over the age of 65 have Alzheimer's. As many as five in ten people over the age of 85 have Alzheimer's. Through research, we are learning more about how the brain is affected by Alzheimer's. We do not yet know how to prevent or cure it.

There is some promising research that indicates that in the early stages the symptoms of Alzheimer's can be controlled with drugs. Ask you doctor about the drugs that might be suitable for a love one with Alzheimer's disease. People who start treatment with these drugs early may keep memory and thinking skills longer. Also, treatment may help people keep doing their daily tasks longer, therefore allowing them to be more independent longer.

There is hope for those of you who have Alzheimer's and h
for your love ones. Even if medication is not right for you or yo
family member, you can make the most of the years you have. Make
sure that your affairs are in order and make a living will so that your
love ones are not confused about your wishes. Also appoint a
guardian while you can. It makes it easier on you and your love ones.

T IS GOUT?

..D said unto Satan, Hast thou considered my servant Job,
..ere is] none like him in the earth, a perfect and an upright man,
..e that feareth God, and escheweth evil? and still he holdeth fast his
integrity, although thou movedest me against him, to destroy him
without cause.

ର~ Job 2:3

Gout is the most common form of arthritis, which is a fancy word for swollen, painful joints. With gout you usually go to bed feeling normal and wake up with pain and swelling. Gout usually affects only one or two joints at a time — most often the feet and toes. The ball of the big toe is the commonest site. Without treatment the attack subsides in a week or so and when patients first develop gout there may be intervals of many months or even years between attacks. As time goes by, these tend to become more frequent and more severe and eventually many joints may be involved, sometimes all at the same time. At this stage, a state of chronic or continuous joint disease may develop with progressive joint damage, disability and crippling (chronic gout). Gout affects mostly men and is very rare in women until after menopause when it is quite often seen.

Uric acid is a chemical which is a natural part of the normal breaking down and building up of food and body tissues. The level in the blood can be measured and shows how much there is in the body overall. When you have gout, uric acid is not broken down and eliminated normally and builds up in the joints of your ankle, foot and big toe. There are many things that can cause a build up of uric acid:

- Higher than normal levels of uric acid can be part of the inherited make-up of some families
- Obesity
- High alcohol intake
- Some of the drugs used to treat high blood pressure

- Less commonly, longstanding kidney disease may result in high blood levels of uric acid.

Anti-inflammatory drugs (NSAIDs) can be very effective to treat the pain of swelling of gout. With effective treatment the attack may be controlled within 12–24 hours and treatment need not be continued after a few days. Rest and elevation of the part involved and a fluid intake increased by an extra four or five glasses of water a day are also important. Drugs used for the acute attack have no effect on reducing uric acid levels. People with gout also have to have their high levels of gout treated. There are drugs that can lower the uric acid but these drugs have no effect on the actual attacks of acute gout and they must be taken on a continuous and long term basis. The dose of the drug that lowers uric acid must be adjusted by repeated checks on the blood level of uric acid before a permanent maintenance dose can be decided on. Once the uric acid is down within normal limits, the patient should remain free from gout provided the drug is continued. Some drugs work by increasing elimination via the kidneys and others by blocking uric acid formation.

It is also very important for patients beginning such drugs to realize that for the first few months of treatment, gouty attacks can become more severe and frequent. This is usually controlled by taking one or two tablets a day of an additional drug for at least several months and if any acute attacks do appear they must be treated in the usual way and the long-term medicines continued.

108. DO YOU HAVE GALL BLADDER DISEASE?

For their vine [is] of the vine of Sodom, and of the fields of Gomorrah:
their grapes [are] grapes of gall, their clusters [are] bitter:

☙ Deuteronomy 32:32

The gall bladder is the organ that helps you digest food. It makes bile which is needed to break down the foods we eat, especially fats. Gallbladder disease is a common condition that mainly affects women, although men can suffer, too. The symptoms vary widely from discomfort to severe pain which mainly begins after food is eaten. In severe cases the patient can suffer from jaundice, nausea and fever. The most common reason for gallbladder disease is gallstones.

Gallstones are solid stones formed in the gall bladder from cholesterol, bile salts and calcium. They can vary in size from a few millimeters to a few centimeters. Gallstones are formed when bile contains too much cholesterol. The excess cholesterol forms crystals from which gallstones are made.

Gallstones are seen in all age groups but they are rare in the young. The possibility of developing gallstones increases with age. The following groups are considered to be at increased risk:

- People who have relatives with gallstones.
- People who are obese or overweight.
- People with a high blood cholesterol levels.
- Women who take drugs containing estrogen-for example birth control pills with estrogen.
- People with diseases such as chronic intestinal inflammation (Crohn's Disease and ulcerative colitis).

It is thought that approximately two thirds of patients will have no trouble at all from their gallstones and only one third of patients will, at some time, experience symptoms. These symptoms can be extremely variable but can present in the following ways:

- sporadic pains in the middle of the upper abdomen, or just below the ribs on the right side.
- the pain may spread to the right shoulder or between the shoulder blades.
- the pain can be accompanied by nausea and vomiting and sometimes excessive flatulence or gas.
- the attack can last from a few minutes to two to three hours before getting better.
- the frequency and severity of attacks is very variable.
- attacks can be triggered by eating fatty foods such as chocolate, cheese or pastry.

When you experience symptoms like those described above, it is known as a gallbladder attack or cholecystitis. The gallbladder is reacting to the stones in it. If you develop fever with these symptoms it is a medical emergency and you should seek care from your physician right away. You will probably have to go to the hospital and have IV antibiotics. Sometimes the stones in the gallbladder can block the opening of the gallbladder and restrict the flow of bile. When this happens you will not only have the symptoms described above, but your eyes and skin can turn yellow or jaundiced as well.

The best treatment for gallbladder disease is to eliminate the things in you diet and life style that cause the stones to form. A diet low in cholesterol and fats will greatly help you to reduce the chance of developing gallstones and having the ones there become smaller or dissolve. This will also help you to lose weight. If the symptoms become too severe or you develop an acute attack with fever you will probably have to have surgery to remove your gallbladder. What you want to avoid is having one of those stones block the emptying of the gallbladder because a blocked bile duct tube can be life threatening.

You are in complete control of whether you develop gallbladder disease by avoiding those foods that can cause you to develop stones. Gallbladder disease is not a disease you want to have, so eat responsibly.

109. WHEN SHOULD I GET A COLONOSCOPY?

And thou [shalt have] great sickness by disease of thy bowels, until thy bowels fall out by reason of the sickness day by day.

ᴈ 2 Chronicles 21:15

A colonoscope is a flexible tube that can be placed into your rectum that allows the physician to see the inside of your large bowel. The test procedure is known as colonoscopy. Colonoscopy lets the physician look inside your entire large intestine, from the lowest part, the rectum, all the way up through the colon to the lower end of the small intestine. The procedure is used to look for early signs of cancer in the colon and rectum. It is also used to diagnose the causes of unexplained changes in bowel habits. Colonoscopy enables the physician to see inflamed tissue, abnormal growths, ulcers, and bleeding.

For the procedure, you will lie on your left side on the examining table. You will probably be given pain medication and a mild sedative to keep you comfortable and to help you relax during the exam. The physician will insert a long, flexible, lighted tube into your rectum and slowly guide it into your colon. The scope transmits an image of the inside of the colon, so the physician can carefully examine the lining of the colon. The scope bends, so the physician can move it around the curves of your colon. You may be asked to change position occasionally to help the physician move the scope. The scope also blows air into your colon, which inflates the colon and helps the physician see better.

If anything abnormal is seen in your colon, like a polyp or inflamed tissue, the physician can remove all or part of it using tiny instruments passed through the scope. That tissue (biopsy) is then sent to a lab for testing. If there is bleeding in the colon, the physician can pass a laser, heater probe, or electrical probe, or can inject special medicines through the scope and use it to stop the bleeding.

Bleeding and puncture of the colon are possible complications of colonoscopy. However, such complications are uncommon.

Colonoscopy takes 30 to 60 minutes. The sedative and pain medicine should keep you from feeling much discomfort during the exam. You will need to remain at the colonoscopy facility for 1 to two hours until the sedative wears off.

Preparation

Your colon must be completely empty for the colonoscopy to be thorough and safe. To prepare for the procedure you may have to follow a liquid diet for 1 to three days beforehand. A liquid diet means fat-free bouillon or broth, strained fruit juice, water, plain coffee, plain tea, or diet soda. Gelatin or popsicles in any color but red may also be eaten. You will also take one of several types of laxatives the night before the procedure. Also, you must arrange for someone to take you home afterward—you will not be allowed to drive because of the sedatives. Your physician may give you other special instructions. Inform your physician of any medical conditions or medications that you take before the colonoscopy.

110. THE FACTS ABOUT MRSA— METHICILLIN RESISTANT STAPHYLOCOCCAL AUREAUS INFECTION

According to the Centers of Disease Control and Prevention (CDC) Staphylococcus aureus, commonly referred to as Staph, are bacteria that live normally on your skin and in your nose. Staph can occasionally cause infection and is the most common form of skin infections in America. Most pimples and boils are caused by Staph and most heal by themselves. There is a kind of Staph infection running rampant in hospitals and now in the community—this Staph is known as Methicillin Resistant Staphylococcus or MRSA. Over the last 50 years this common bacteria has become smart enough not to be affected by treatment with this simple penicillin-like antibiotic. Most scientist think it's because we as Americans used too much Penicillin to treat diseases and in return made the friendly bacteria that live normally on our skin resistant to the penicillin family of antibiotics.

The CDC has an increase in reports of infections in healthy adults and children with MRSA. When the MRSA breaks through our first defense, the skin, it can infect us through the blood to infect our bones, lungs and other organs. MRSA can also cause very serious skin infections. One of the dangers of being in the hospital is that you will get a skin or wound infection with MRSA. If you live in cramped quarters with a lot of people, you can get MRSA as well. If you share needles with other IV drug users you can get MRSA. MRSA is almost always spread by direst physical contact of an infected person or from contact with surfaces such as towels, sheets, wound dressings, clothes, workout areas, sports equipment, or shoes, from someone with MRSA.

To avoid getting MRSA follow this simple rule: practice good hygiene and always wash your hands.